ISPOR Taxonomy of Patient Registries: Classification, Characteristics and Terms

ISPOR Taxonomy of Patient Registries: Classification, Characteristics and Terms

Editor-in-Chief

Dimitris Polygenis, PharmD

Assistant Editors

Diana Frame, MPH

Kirsten Hall Long, PhD

John McCormick, PhD

Section Editors

Chris Blanchette, PhD, MS, MA

Eric Gemmen, MA

Shital Kamble, PhD, MS

Leanne Larson, MHA

Managing Editor

Elizabeth Molsen, RN

LAWRENCEVILLE, NJ

ISPOR Taxonomy of Patient Registries: Classification, Characteristics and Terms

Published by
International Society for Pharmacoeconomics and Outcomes Research (ISPOR)
505 Lawrence Square Blvd. South
Lawrenceville, NJ 08648 USA
Tel: 1-609-586-4981 | Toll Free: 1-800-992-0643
Fax: 1-609-586-4982
Email: info@ispor.org | Website: www.ispor.org

Ordering information is available by calling ISPOR at 609-586-4981, or visit the ISPOR website at www.ispor.org.

Library of Congress Control Number 2013934674
ISBN 978-0-9743289-4-2

Printed in the United States of America.

Contents

Contributors . . . vii
Acknowledgements . . . ix
About ISPOR . . . xi
Introduction . . . 3

SECTION I: Patient Registry Definition and Characteristics . . . 5

SECTION II: Design, Development and Implementation of Patient Registries . . . 15

Registry Purpose . . . 17
Scientific Objectives . . . 17
Rationale . . . 18
Research Participants . . . 19
Research Questions . . . 20
Validity . . . 21
- Internal Validity . . . 22
- External Validity . . . 23
Study Limitations . . . 24
Transparency . . . 25
Reproducibility . . . 26
Outcomes/End Points . . . 27
Outcomes/End Points . . . 27
Efficacy . . . 28
- Clinical Effectiveness . . . 28
- Comparative Effectiveness . . . 29
Safety . . . 31
- Adverse Events . . . 31
- Passive Safety Surveillance . . . 32
- Active Safety Surveillance . . . 33
- Reporting of Safety Outcomes . . . 34
Other Types of Outcomes . . . 35
- Health-Related Quality of Life (HRQOL) Outcomes . . . 35
- Direct Costs . . . 37
- Indirect Costs . . . 39
- Cost-Effectiveness and Cost Utility . . . 40
- Compliance/Adherence . . . 41
- Persistence . . . 43
- Treatment Satisfaction . . . 44

General Study Design . . . 46
Retrospective . . . 46
Case-Control Study . . . 47
Prospective . . . 48
- Interventional . . . 48
- Noninterventional/Observational . . . 49
Cohort Study . . . 50
Usual Care . . . 51
Standard of Care . . . 52
Treatment Guidelines/Consensus . . . 53
Stakeholders . . . 54
Primary Stakeholder . . . 54
Secondary Stakeholders . . . 54
Governance and Oversight . . . 55
Scientific Advisory Board (SAB) . . . 56
Data Ownership and Access Rights . . . 57
Ethics and Privacy . . . 59
Belmont Report (Public Law 93-348 [1974], Title II) . . . 59
- Respect for Persons . . . 60
- Beneficence . . . 61
- Justice . . . 62
Informed Consent . . . 62
Common Rule . . . 63
Institutional Review Board (IRB)/Ethical Committee Approval . . . 64
Council for International Organization of Medical Sciences (CIOMS) International Guidelines for Ethical Review of Epidemiological Studies . . . 66
Declaration of Helsinki . . . 66
International Conference on Harmonization (ICH): Good Clinical Practice (GCP) . . . 67
US Food and Drug Administration (FDA) Regulations . . . 68
Conflict of Interest . . . 69
Data Privacy and Committees . . . 70
Deidentified Information . . . 71
Data Protection . . . 73
Privacy Rule/US Health Insurance Portability and Accountability Act (HIPAA) . . . 74
Implementation and Operational Considerations . . . 76
Size . . . 76
Budget . . . 77
Feasibility . . . 78
Standard Operating Procedures (SOPs) . . . 79
Pretesting/Pilot testing . . . 80
Study Population . . . 81
Sampling . . . 82
Comparison Group . . . 83

- Internal Comparator . . . 83
- External Comparator . . . 83
- Historical Comparator . . . 83
- Matched Control . . . 84
Duration of Observation . . . 85
Core Dataset . . . 86
Data: Sources, Elements, Capture and Quality Assurance . . . 87
Primary Data Sources . . . 87
Secondary Data Sources . . . 88
- Medical Charts . . . 88
- Electronic Health Records (EHRs) . . . 88
- Institutional or Organizational Databases . . . 88
- Administrative Databases . . . 88
- Birth and Death Records . . . 89
- Census Databases . . . 89
- Existing Registries . . . 89
Data Domains . . . 90
- Exposures . . . 90
- Outcomes . . . 90
- Patient . . . 90
- Diagnostics . . . 91
- Provider . . . 91
- Environmental . . . 91
- Adverse Events . . . 91
Data Definitions . . . 92
Data Capture/Collection . . . 93
Instrument or Scale Validation . . . 93
- Content Validity . . . 94
- Construct Validity . . . 94
- Criterion Validity . . . 94
- Reliability . . . 94
- Responsiveness . . . 95
- Interpretability/Clinical Meaningfulness . . . 95
Case Report Forms (CRFs) . . . 96
Mode of Administration . . . 97
Electronic Data Capture . . . 98
Database Build . . . 99
Clinical Data Standards . . . 100
Data Quality Assurance . . . 101
Edit Checks/Specifications . . . 102
Data Cleaning . . . 103
On-site Monitoring . . . 103
Centralized or Remote Monitoring . . . 104

Site Support and Data Management ... 106
Site Identification and Recruitment ... 106
Site Start-up ... 107
Site Training ... 108
Regulatory Documents ... 109
Investigator Meetings ... 109
Patient Recruitment ... 110
Patient Retention ... 111
Recruitment and Retention Tools ... 112
Site Reimbursement ... 113
Patient Honoraria ... 114
Loss to Follow-up ... 114
Enrollment Log/Screening Log ... 116
Performance Measure ... 117
Help Desk ... 117
Clinical Research Associate (CRA) ... 118
Source Document Verification (SDV) ... 119
Query Resolution ... 120
Close-out ... 122
Site Close-out ... 122
Data Transfer ... 122
Record Retention and Database Archiving ... 123
Evaluating and Ensuring Registry Quality ... 125
Agency for Healthcare Research and Quality Guidance for Registries ... 125
European Medicines Agency's (EMA) Guidance on HRQOL ... 126
European Network of Centres for Pharmacoepidemiology and Pharmacovigilance (ENCePP) ... 126
Guidelines for Good Pharmacoepidemiology Practices (GPP) ... 127
Guidance for Industry: Good Pharmacovigilance Practices and Pharmacoepidemiological Assessment ... 128
Guidelines for Evaluating Public Health Surveillance Systems ... 129
Swedish Association of the Pharmaceutical Industry (LIF): Rules for Noninterventional Studies ... 130
Good Research Practice Considerations ... 131
CONSORT (Consolidated Standard of Reporting Trials) ... 131
GRACE (Good ReseArch for Comparative Effectiveness) ... 132
STROBE (STrengthening the Reporting of OBservational studies in Epidemiology) ... 133

SECTION III: Analysis and Reporting of Patient Registry Data ... 135

Analysis ... 137
Analysis Plan ... 137
Statistical Inference and Hypothesis Testing ... 138
Confidence Intervals ... 138

Hypothesis Testing and P-values 140
Statistical Significance Under Large Sample Sizes 141
Multiplicity Adjustments 142
Available Variables for Analyses 146
- Quantitative Variables 146
- Continuous 146
- Count 146
- Categorical Variables 147
- Nominal/Qualitative/Dichotomous 147
- Ordinal 147
- Outcome(s) of Interest 147
- Independent Variables 148
- Confounders/Covariates 148
Missing Observations 150
- Missing Completely at Random (MCAR) 150
- Missing at Random (MAR) 150
- Missing Not at Random (MNAR) 151
Strategies for Handling Missing Observations 151
- Strategies when Data is MCAR 152
- Strategies when Data is MAR 153
- Strategies when Data is MNAR 153
Timing of Analyses 155
Interim Analysis 155
Post Hoc Analyses 156
Sensitivity Analyses 156
Analysis Techniques 158
Summary Statistics for Quantitative Variables 158
Summary Statistics for Qualitative Variables 160
Statistical Inference and Tests 161
Analyzing 2 or More Variables 162
Student's T-tests 163
Wilcoxon Rank-Sum Test 164
Chi-square Test 165
Analysis of Variance (ANOVA) 166
Ordinary Least Squares (OLS) Models 166
Logistic/Logit and Probit Models 167
- Ordinal Logistic/Logit and Ordinal Probit Models 168
- Multinomial Logistic/Logit and Multinomial Probit Models 168
Poisson Model 169
Negative Binomial Model 170
Generalized Estimating Equations 171
Cox-Proportional Hazards Regression Model 172
2-Part Model 173
Multilevel Modeling 175

- Population-Average Model 175
- Random-Effects Model 176
- Fixed-Effects Model 176
Generalized Linear Model 178
Risk-Adjustment Techniques 180
- Charlson Comorbidity Index 180
- Adaptations of Charlson Index: Deyo/Charlson Adaptation, Romano/Charlson Adaptation, and D'Hoore/Charlson Implementation 180
- Elixhauser Comorbid Disease Adjustment Method 180
Treatment Effect/Effect Size 182
Selection Bias 183
Propensity Score Matching 184
Treatment Effects Models and Instrumental Variables 185
Jackknife 187
Bootstrap 188
Systematic Reviews/Meta-analysis 189
- Systematic Reviews 189
- Meta-analysis 189
Reporting and Dissemination of Registry-Based Studies 193
Reporting Requirements 193
Publication 193
Authorship 194
Peer Review 195
Publication Bias 196
Overlapping Publications 197

Acronym Reference List 199
About the Editors 201
Index 207

Contributors

Elisa Alfieri, BA, MHA, Business Development Specialist, Lovelace Respiratory Research Institute, Kannapolis, NC, USA

Christopher M. Blanchette, PhD, MS, MA, Research Associate Professor, Department of Public Health Sciences, University of North Carolina - Charlotte, Charlotte, NC, USA

Maznah Dahlui, MD, MPH, PhD, Lecturer, University of Malaya, Kuala Lumpur, Malaysia

Donatus Ekwueme, PhD, Senior Health Economist, US Centers for Disease Control and Prevention, Division of Cancer Prevention, Sandy Springs, GA, USA

John Ellison, MS, Senior Manager, Health Economics Research and Medical Writing, Acclarent, Menlo Park, CA, USA

Alex Exuzides, PhD, Director, ICON Late Phase & Outcomes Research, San Francisco, CA, USA

Claudio Faria, PharmD, MPH, Director, Health Outcomes and Economics Research, Eisai, Inc., Quincy, MA, USA

Lauren Farmer, BS, MSc, Project Manager, Lovelace Respiratory Research Institute, Albuquerque, NM, USA

Diana Frame, MPH, Founder, Frame Research, Brooklyn, NY, USA

Paula Funk-Orsini, PhD, President, Arete Medical Outcomes Research, New York, NY, USA

Carl Gibbons, BSc, Group Health Economics Manager (Specialty Care), Roche Products Limited, Welwyn, Garden City, England, UK

Eric Gemmen, MA, Senior Director, Medical Affairs, Epidemiology & Outcomes Research, Quintiles, Inc., Rockville, MD, USA

Matthew Gordon, BA, Senior Director, Observational Research, PharmaNet, Deerfield, IL, USA

Joao Guerra, MD, MBA, Researcher, National School of Public Health, Lisboa, Portugal

Kirsten Hall Long, PhD, Senior Health Economist, K. Long Consulting, LLC, St. Paul, MN, USA

Elizabeth Hernberg Stahl, MSc, Senior Research Scientist, United Biosource Corporation, London, England, UK

Nadja Hoebel, MSc, Manager Registry and Health Outcomes, Kendle GmbH, Munich, Germany

Joanna Lis, PhD, MSc, Director of Public Affairs and Market Access Dept., Sanofi-Aventis Sp. z o.o., Warsaw, Poland

Shital Kamble, PhD, MS, MBA, BPharm, Senior Outcomes Research Manager, Scientific Affairs, Real World & Late Phase Research, Quintiles Outcome, Rockville, MD, USA

Leanne Larson, MHA, Vice President, Evidence Development, PAREXEL International, Wilmette, IL, USA

Yvonne Lis, PhD, Consultant, PAREXEL International, Uxbridge, England, UK

Steven Lister, MA, BA, Senior Health Economic & Outcomes Research Manager, Bristol-Myers Squibb, Uxbridge, UK

Neal Mantick, BS, MSc, Senior Director, Observational Research, PAREXEL International, Waltham, MA, USA

John McCormick, PhD, Senior Consultant, McKesson Specialty, McKesson Canada, Toronto, ON, CA

Elizabeth Molsen RN, Director, Scientific & Health Policy Initiatives, ISPOR, Lawrenceville, NJ, USA

Chris Pashos, PhD, Vice President, United BioSource Corporation, Lexington, MA, USA

Anuprita Patkar, PhD, Associate Director, Ethicon, Princeton, NJ, USA

Dimitris Polygenis, PharmD, Vice President & General Manager, Pharmaceutical Solutions, McKesson Canada, Toronto, ON, CA

Matthew Reaney, MSc, BSc, Global Health Outcomes Scientist, Endocrine, Eli Lilly, Windlesham, UK

Gabriel Sandblom, MD, PhD, Ward Physician, Department of Surgery, University Hospital - Lund, Lund, Sweden

Adithya Sivaraju, MD, Neurologist, University of Medicine and Dentistry in New Jersey, Newark, NJ, USA

Kathryn Starzyk, MSc, BA, Director of Scientific Affairs, Outcome Sciences, Outcome Sciences, MA, USA

Sally Thompson, PhD, MSc, Outcomes Research Director, Pfizer Ltd, Surrey, UK

Grace Wang - Leung, MPH, International l Payer Strategy Leader, Genentech, Inc., South San Francisco, CA, USA

Acknowledgements

It is with much appreciation that I would like to thank John McCormick for his significant contributions in the final stretch, Elizabeth Molsen for her stewardship, and my family, Lynda, Christian and Michael; without their patience and support this book would not be a reality.

Dimitris Polygenis, PharmD
Editor-in-Chief

It is my pleasure to thank the editorial team for their diligence, dedication and perseverance during this challenging process to complete the book on deadline: Editor-in-Chief, Dimitris Polygenis, for his leadership and the assistant editors: John McCormick, Diana Frame and Kirsten Hall Long. This book would not be ready for the ISPOR 18th Annual International Meeting in New Orleans without the 4 of you.

Many thanks go to the section editors: Shital Kamble, Chris Blanchette, Leanne Larson and Eric Gemmen for their hard work, time, and energy in bringing the book to this point; and finally, Bethann Carbone at ExpressIt Media who worked many long hours and late nights to bring all the pieces together into a solid publication.

To my colleagues: Nadia Naaman, Randa Eldessouki, Rebecca Corey, and Marilyn Dix Smith—thank you for your support during this five year process. It is much appreciated. I also want to thank Maria Swift for organizational assistance; Eden McConnell for excellent proofreading; Steve Priori for assisting with publication; and Susie Henkel for her graphic artist wizardry on the striking cover design and promotional pieces.

On a personal note, thank you to my parents and grandmother for their love and support throughout my career and education and to Adrian for his love, support and patience during the publication of 5 task force reports and 2 books.

Elizabeth Molsen, RN
Managing Editor

About ISPOR

Founded in 1995, the International Society for Pharmacoeconomics and Outcomes Research (ISPOR) is a nonprofit, international, educational, and scientific organization that facilitates the translation of outcomes research into useful information for health care decisions at all levels. ISPOR communicates health care information through several channels: its 3 journals, *Value in Health*, *Value in Health Regional Issues*, and *ISPOR CONNECTIONS*; annual meetings, congresses, and biennial regional conferences, as well as ISPOR's educational program that includes distance learning, short courses, and continuing education.

In addition, ISPOR provides tools for health care decision makers, educators, payers, researchers, students and patients. ISPOR has published more than 50 ISPOR Good Practices for Outcomes Research Reports, consensus guidelines on key outcomes research methods. The Society has also produced the ISPOR Research Digest, a searchable database of nearly 30,000 abstracts and presentations from ISPOR meetings; the ISPOR Global Health Care Systems Road Map; the International Digest of Databases; and web-based questionnaires on assessing evidence in observational, modeling and other types of research studies. All of these are available to the public on the ISPOR website (www.ispor.org).

ISPOR has over 7,000 active members from more than 100 countries around the world. In addition, ISPOR's 64 Regional Chapters expand ISPOR's reach to over 13,000 members.

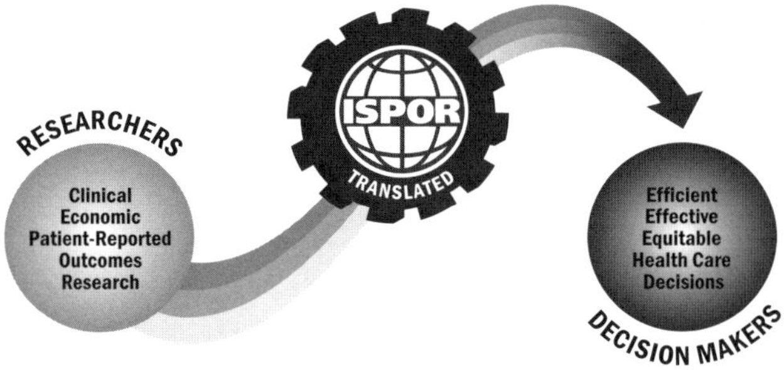

ISPOR promotes outcomes research and its use in evidence-based health care decisions

Introduction

The growing importance of registries and their increasing prominence in defining the health management environment prompted members of the International Society for Pharmacoeconomics and Outcomes Research (ISPOR) Patient Registry Special Interest Group to develop the *ISPOR Taxonomy of Patient Registries: Classification, Characteristics and Terms* (*Taxonomy*). More than 30 ISPOR members with relevant experience (patient registry, clinical trial, pharmaceutical and/or outcomes research experience), working in academia, governmental institutions, research organizations, or the pharmaceutical and device industries from around the world contributed to the expert opinion incorporated in this consensus handbook.

The *Taxonomy* is for decision makers, clinicians, students and outcomes research practitioners. It attempts to define a unifying prospective plan for registry data collection and analysis to guide in the design and execution of effective registry-based studies. It will assist the reader in registry development, the use of registry data for analysis, and the incorporation of registry data results in decision making, literature reviews or cost models.

It is a user-friendly encyclopedia of terms as well as a reference book. The *Taxonomy* defines terms used in the design, development and implementation of registries, as well as those used in the analysis, reporting and publishing of registry data. Each term includes a brief definition, a broader explanation, the associated values and uses, and concludes with a discussion of issues or conflicts related to the term. While many aspects of registries overlap with traditional clinical research, the book will attempt to highlight differences, key issues and considerations.

This book is divided into 3 sections: **Section I: Patient Registry Definition and Characteristics**; **Section II: Design, Development and Implementation of Patient Registries** and **Section III: Analysis and Reporting of Patient Registry Data**.

Section I: Patient Registry Definition and Characteristics provides an overview of patient registries. Currently, there is no consensus on what defines a patient registry. This section delves into universal patient registry features and what distinguishes registries from other observational research studies. By comparing and contrasting the elements common to clinical trials and illustrating their relevance to patient registries, a framework is established to define registries' place in the outcomes research field.

Section II: Design, Development and Implementation explains how to establish an effective registry and how to ensure that high-quality data is generated. It opens with the registry's purpose and describes the types of outcomes that a registry can generate. The mechanics of initiating a registry are outlined in terms of site selection and management, patient recruitment, potential data sources, and data capture and management. Recommendations on registry design, operations, stakeholders, ethics and good practices are included.

Section III: Analysis and Reporting of Patient Registry Data describes how to effectively analyze data that has been generated by registries. It explains the different approaches to data analysis and how to identify and deal with commonly encountered biases in registry design. The section opens with development of an analysis plan. Recommendations are made on statistical models that can be used to identify and quantify correlations between patient parameters and clinical and economic outcomes, as well as how to demonstrate significant data trends. Dealing with missing observations is addressed, as well as potential differences in recruited patients.

Finally, this section describes the steps involved in effectively reporting and disseminating the results of registry studies. The authors hope that this approach will strengthen the validity of outcomes based on registry data and minimize the potential sources of bias.

The goal of this book is to go beyond simply terms. The terminology sections in ISPOR's *Taxonomy* provide an overview of patient registries from start to finish, leading the reader chronologically through the process of registry design, development, and implementation. Terminology on registry data is organized similarly, with initiation of the analysis plan, through reporting and dissemination of registry-based studies. In this manner, the reader will understand all the steps involved and be able to better plan registry development and research. The *Taxonomy* will contribute to standardizing the language used in the patient registry field and improve registry-based research.

SECTION I

Patient Registry Definition and Characteristics

The *ISPOR Taxonomy of Patient Registries: Classification, Characteristics and Terms* attempts to define appropriate language for patient registry research: both the establishment of registries (design, development, and implementation) and how the generated data can be effectively utilized (analysis and reporting). In addition, as there is no broad consensus as to what defines a patient registry, the book highlights important registry characteristics and attempts to standardize patient registry terminology.

For the purposes of this book, **a *patient registry* is defined as a prospective observational study of subjects with certain shared characteristics, which collects ongoing and supporting data over time on well-defined outcomes of interest for analysis and reporting**. In layman's terms, registries are designed to observe and collect information on health care experiences and interventions that would normally be part of routine clinical practice.

Registries are intended to investigate a complementary set of issues around a clinical scenario that cannot be properly evaluated or assessed in the artificial environment of a traditional controlled trial. They are often designed and launched to observe *real-world* treatment(s) and related clinical outcomes among patients with a specific disease, or among patients receiving a specific treatment. However, even in the case of registries designed to study a specific medical treatment, the registry protocol does not dictate specific treatments, assessments, procedures or tests, as commonly seen in controlled clinical trial studies. Thus, they are considered noninterventional in nature as they merely *observe* clinical practice.

REGISTRY CHARACTERISTICS

The Phase III randomized controlled trial (RCT)[1] is a pivotal component in the approval process for new drugs. It provides vital information on the efficacy and safety of a new medication. However, due to strict patient-inclusion criteria, limited observation periods, and protocol-driven tests and procedures, the observed drug efficacy in a RCT may not reflect the actual effectiveness or safety of the drug when it is used in real-world clinical settings. Assessment of real-world safety, including rare events that would be unlikely to occur in a sample size of a typical Phase III study, is often a driving factor for the establishment of registries. A patient registry may be required or requested by regulatory agencies. As a result, postmarketing observational studies are becoming increasingly important.

Payers, as well as regulators, may require additional data on how a specific drug is utilized in clinical practice or data on the identification of the barriers preventing

1. A clinical trial is a specific type of scientific experiment that include patients (commonly referred to as subjects) meeting specific inclusion and exclusion criteria and following a precise protocol. The acronym, RCT, is often used synonymously for randomized clinical trial and randomized controlled trial; the latter considered to be the gold-standard. In a randomized controlled trial, the control group could include subjects receiving placebo (no treatment) or subjects receiving usual or standard care. In a randomized clinical or randomized comparative trial, the comparison is of multiple treatment groups with each other.

the drug from showing its maximum effectiveness in this environment. These impediments are usually a complex mix of clinical and nonclinical parameters, which can include patient noncompliance with therapy, inappropriate prescribing by physicians, secondary consequences of an increased negative impact of the prescribed therapy on patients' health-related quality of life (HRQOL) and the inability of all patients to successfully gain access to a specific drug.

Payers may also be interested in learning how a new medication impacts the overall burden of a specific disease and how this, in turn, impacts broader societal health care resources and costs. These broader outcomes cannot be accurately assessed through a Phase III trial. Even postmarketing Phase IV studies can be limited in their ability to capture all relevant real-world outcomes.

Registries provide an alternative way to quantify these outcomes in a postmarketing environment and can be used to assess broader aspects of health care. Registries can also be used to assess nonhealth-related issues and to address reimbursement issues related to a specific drug, drug class or disease that may impact a patient's ability to access effective treatment.

Unlike controlled clinical trials in which the trial's protocol stipulates patient inclusion and exclusion criteria to minimize bias and promote internal data validity, real-world registries typically have heterogeneous patient enrollment. Comorbid conditions and the use of concomitant medications are more prevalent among registry patients. As a result, data from registries is often used to complement prior clinical trial data by focusing on external generalizability within the more complicated real-world treatment setting. Some of the outcomes that can be generated from registries are summarized in Table 1, as are the unique differences between registries and RCTs.

Registries differ from other postmarketing observational studies, too. Patient registries do <u>not</u> follow a study protocol. Study protocols modify real-world clinical practice. Protocol-driven treatment algorithms, protocol-mandated physician visits, or specific patient assessments distinguish other types of observational studies from registries. For example, Phase IIIb to Phase IV studies can include a defined treatment or medical intervention. In addition, they can be conducted as RCTs, with patient populations randomized to different therapies. If there is any kind of protocol-driven allocation of patients to a specific assessment schedule or procedure, the study is no longer observational and is not considered a registry.

As a result of their patient heterogeneity, generalizability and unique, prospective, noninterventional design, patient registries are increasingly used to evaluate disease-related resource utilization, drug class utilization, health and disease management and patient reported outcomes (eg, patient-satisfaction assessments), as well as clinical outcomes, safety surveillance and risk assessment. (see Table 2).

Common registry design features, the type of clinical, economic and safety outcomes generated and how the data can be effectively utilized, are also summarized in Table 2. In addition, this table lists the potential sponsors of different

TABLE 1: Comparison of Registries with Randomized Controlled Trials (RCTs)

Study Parameter	Registries	RCTs
Methods	Do not require a comparator or placebo; tend to reflect typical care	The only truly controlled design, though the comparator or placebo may not always be clinically relevant
Randomization	Is not used to assign patients to different treatment groups	Is used to assign patients to different treatment groups to ensure outcome is related to treatment and not other causes
Double-Blind Placebo Control	Not possible to incorporate	Compares similar patient groups with respect to both known and unknown factors, and ensures similar treatment expectations
Outcomes	May be generalizable to a wide range of patients. May have more external validity	Specific to the patient treatment group being studied Focus is more on internal validity Generalizable to different groups
	More likely to represent real-world outcomes	Can only be associated with the patient and treatment group dictated in the study
Treatment	Evaluate care as it is provided in a real-world setting	Treatment is assigned via a protocol
Practicality	May be more practical, eg, for a very rare disease with small patient numbers	May be impractical to conduct, eg, in the case of a very rare disease when timely patient recruitment may be difficult
Ethics	May be the only ethical solution if RCT not ethical	May not be ethically acceptable
Time Period	Can be used to observe very long-term outcomes	May be impractical or not feasible for observing very long-term outcomes
Confounding	Due to patient selection, varying treatment patterns, and differences in compliance, can generate treatment-outcome associations that are not necessarily causal	Usually have very similar groups before treatment, and dictate treatment and clinical procedures to minimize confounding
Registration	Difficult to require registration	Can be registered to prevent selective reporting
Patients	Can involve large numbers of patients	Involves limited number of participants
	Often involve *typical* patients seen in a real-world setting	Typically involves a *pure* group of patients, through use of inclusion and exclusion criteria, that may not be representative of real-world *typical* patients

TABLE 2: Uses of Patient Registries

Registry Type	Design	Evaluation Measurement	Application/Use	Sponsors
Simple Cohort	• Prospective • Noninterventional • Sample based • Collection of information in a population that shares common exposure	• Clinical outcomes, eg, morbidity, mortality	• Pregnancy registry • Determine association/correlation between exposure and outcome	• Epidemiologists • Public health • Clinicians
Outcomes	• Prospective • Noninterventional • Population based • Collection of information in a population	• Clinical outcomes, eg, morbidity, mortality	• Understand natural history of a patient cohort sharing common characteristics, eg, social science research, population-based research, epidemiological research • Examples: mortality, literacy, access to medical care, etc.	• Epidemiologists • Policy makers • Governments • Public health • Academia
Safety Surveillance	• Prospective • Noninterventional • Sample based • Collection of information in patients receiving a common intervention	• Adverse events • Unexpected adverse events • Serious adverse events	• Support product registration • Conduct postmarketing surveillance (real-world setting) • Identify *signals*	• Manufacturers • Regulators • Clinicians

continued on next page >

< continued from previous page

Registry Type	Design	Evaluation Measurement	Application/Use	Sponsors
Risk Management	• Prospective • Noninterventional although limited to a specific intervention • Population based • Use one or more tools to meet goal(s) • May collect information beyond FDA-approved labeling	• Clinical outcomes • Safety information and adverse events • Compliance with prescribed management protocols • Impact of tools on ensuring compliance	• Mandated by regulators to meet specific goals and objectives in minimizing known risks while preserving benefits • Assessing product's risk-benefit balance • Developing and evaluating tools to minimize risks while preserving benefits • Making adjustments to risk management tools to further improve risk-benefit balance	• Regulators • Manufacturers
Disease	• Prospective • Noninterventional • Population based • Collects information in a cohort of patients with common disease	• Drug utilization and safety • Clinical outcomes, eg, morbidity, mortality • Resource utilization • Clinical management	• Understand natural history of disease • Identify, compare and evaluate management patterns • Identify *signals* relating to safety, effectiveness and outcomes • Quantify burden of illness, HRQOL • May assist in establishing and benchmarking best practices • Assess screening, identification and monitoring practices • Allow assessment of cost-effectiveness of management practices	• Clinicians • Health policy makers • Public health • Epidemiologists • Payers

continued on next page >

< continued from previous page

Registry Type	Design	Evaluation Measurement	Application/Use	Sponsors
Drug and Drug Class	• Prospective (may include some retrospective data) • Sample based • Collects information on a patient cohort receiving common treatment	• Safety and effectiveness • Clinical outcomes, eg, morbidity and mortality • Resource utilization • Clinical management and add-on therapy	• Postmarketing surveillance • Compare effectiveness to efficacy • Study nonapproved uses • Identify drug-related *signals* • Cost-effectiveness • Willingness to pay • Reimbursement evaluation	• Clinicians • Manufacturers • Regulators • Payers
Management	• Prospective (may include some retrospective data) • Collect information on a common population • Population/Sample based	• Treatment and management patterns • Resource utilization • Clinical and economic outcomes	• Care mapping • Continuous quality improvement • Resource utilization and costing • Burden of illness • Quality of care • Provider performance • Health economic evaluation • Reimbursement evaluation	• Payers • Clinicians • Health policy makers • Health administrators • Academia
Resource Utilization	• Prospective (may include some retrospective data) • Sample based	• Direct costs, eg, medical care, drug use, hospitalization • Productivity costs, eg, absenteeism, productivity	• Burden of illness • Cost of care • Reimbursement evaluation • Health economic evaluations	• Payers • Policy makers • Clinicians • Health administrators • Academia

types of registry-based studies. For a database of existing patient registries, please see the Registry of Patient Registries (RoPR) available on the Agency for Healthcare Research and Quality (AHRQ) website, www.ahrq.gov.

BIBLIOGRAPHY

Gliklich RE, Dreyer NA, eds. *Registries for Evaluating Patient Outcomes: A User's Guide*. 2nd ed. (Prepared by Outcome DEcIDE Center [Outcome Sciences, Inc. d/b/a Outcome] under contract no. HHSA290200500351 T03.) AHRQ Publication No. 10-EHC049. Rockville, MD: Agency for Healthcare Research and Quality; 2010.

Avorn J. In defense of pharmacoepidemiology—embracing the yin and yang of drug research. *N Engl J Med*. 2007;357:2219-2221.

Shrier I, Boivin JF, Steele RJ, et al. Should meta-analyses of interventions include observational studies in addition to randomized controlled trials? A critical examination of underlying principles. *Am J Epidemiol*. 2007;166:1203-1209.

Sankaranarayanan J, Hartman T, Crown W. The role of patient registries. In: Esposito D, ed. *Reliability and Validity of Data Sources for Outcomes Research & Disease and Health Management Programs*. Lawrenceville, NJ: ISPOR; 2013:300-316.

SECTION II

Design, Development and Implementation of Patient Registries

Registry Purpose

Scientific Objectives

BRIEF DEFINITION

A documented statement of specific objectives or goals for the registry. The goals and purpose of a registry are generally set out in a synopsis or protocol.

EXPLANATION

A registry may have a singular focus, or it may serve several purposes. In either case, the overall purpose should be translated into specific objectives or questions to be addressed through the registry. The goals of a registry may relate to basic research (research without immediate clinical application such as observation of the natural history of a disease), evaluation of outcomes associated with different interventions (effectiveness, safety, patient-reported outcomes (PROs), or cost-effectiveness [*see term:* Outcomes/End Points]), assessment of drug utilization patterns and persistence on therapy, issues related to quality assurance (assessing provider performance or adherence to treatment guidelines) or health care improvement (research with the aim of improving health care delivery for patients in the target population) (Table 2).

VALUE AND USE

Clear study objectives are an essential step in defining the appropriate outcome analyses. The content of the data to be collected should be driven by the scientific analyses that are planned for the registry, which in turn are determined by the objectives of the registry.

ISSUES

Sponsors of a registry, such as pharmaceutical manufacturers, may have additional goals beyond scientific objectives (*see term:* Stakeholders). These commercial objectives can include the potential benefit achieved by observing and evaluating real-world treatment patterns, effectiveness and safety, determining resource use associated with a particular intervention, or marketing and provider education goals for new interventions.

Care should be taken to ensure that commercial objectives are clearly separated from scientific objectives; a prospective protocol and analysis plan ensure that scientific objectives do not change over the course of a study. In this way, unfavorable results or undue influence by sponsors do not alter the scientific objectives of the study (*see term:* Analysis Plan).

BIBLIOGRAPHY

Chapter 2. Planning a registry. In: Gliklich RE, Dreyer NA, eds. *Registries for Evaluating Patient Outcomes: A User's Guide*. 2nd ed. (Prepared by Outcome DEcIDE Center [Outcome Sciences, Inc. d/b/a Outcome] under contract no. HHSA290200500351 T03.) AHRQ Publication No. 10-EHC049. Rockville, MD: Agency for Healthcare Research and Quality; 2010:23-52.

von Elm E, Altman DG, Egger M, et al. The Strengthening the Reporting of Observational Studies in Epidemiology (STROBE) statement: guidelines for reporting observational studies. *Epidemiology*. 2007;18:800-804.

Vandenbroucke JP, von Elm E, Altman DG, et al. Strengthening the Reporting of Observational Studies in Epidemiology (STROBE): explanation and elaboration. *Epidemiology*. 2007; 18:805–835.

Dreyer NA, Schneeweiss S, McNeil BJ, et al. GRACE principles: recognizing high-quality observational studies of comparative effectiveness. *Am J Manag Care*. 2010;16:467-471.

Berger ML, Mamdani M, Atkins D, Johnson ML. Good research practices for comparative effectiveness research: defining, reporting and interpreting nonrandomized studies of treatment effects using secondary data sources: the ISPOR Good Research Practices for Retrospective Database Analysis Task Force Report—Part I. *Value Health*. 2009;12:1044-1052.

Sankaranarayanan J, Hartman T, Crown W. The role of patient registries. In: Esposito D, ed. *Reliability and Validity of Data Sources for Outcomes Research & Disease and Health Management Programs*. Lawrenceville, NJ: ISPOR; 2013:300-316.

Rationale

BRIEF DEFINITION

The fundamental reasons for conducting the registry study, collecting the data, and for the analytic techniques chosen.

EXPLANATION

Registries are considered or created for a number of reasons and there is tremendous variability in the size, scope, and resource requirements of the various registries. The rationale for conducting a study in a particular way (such as if the data being sought have already been collected elsewhere, whether or not a registry is the most appropriate means for addressing the research question, and what this registry will add to current knowledge) should be clearly stated in a registry plan or protocol, and reiterated in subsequent reports of study findings.

VALUE AND USE

The rationale answers the *why* question in the context of what is known and not known on the topic to be studied. Reporting the rationale can help the reader understand why the study was designed in a specific way and why specific analytical techniques were used. An explanation of the study rationale is included in the

CONSORT checklist on appropriate reporting of clinical trials (*see term:* Good Research Practice Considerations).

ISSUES

Study rationales are not well documented in some cases; this has been a particular issue with noninferiority analyses. It is important to consider whether or not a registry design is the most appropriate for the clinical question to be answered, and under the relevant logistical and other constraints (*see term:* General Study Design) and these details should be discussed in the rationale.

BIBLIOGRAPHY

Chapter 2. Planning a registry. In: Gliklich RE, Dreyer NA, eds. *Registries for Evaluating Patient Outcomes: A User's Guide.* 2nd ed. (Prepared by Outcome DEcIDE Center [Outcome Sciences, Inc. d/b/a Outcome] under contract no. HHSA290200500351 T03.) AHRQ Publication No. 10-EHC049. Rockville, MD: Agency for Healthcare Research and Quality; 2010:23-52.

Moher D, Schulz KF, Altman D; CONSORT Group (Consolidated Standards of Reporting Trials). The CONSORT statement: revised recommendations for improving the quality of reports of parallel group randomized trials. *JAMA.* 2001;285:1987-1991.

McCaffrey N, Merlin T, Hiller J. Lack of clinical rationale provided for non-inferiority margins. Poster presented at: 3rd Annual Health Technology Assessment International (HTAi) conference; July 3-5, 2006; Adelaide, South Australia.

Research Participants

BRIEF DEFINITION

An individual who has given informed consent to participate in a registry (*see term:* Informed Consent).

EXPLANATION

As registries are observational studies and not investigational trials, the observational unit is generally considered to be the patient or the participant rather than a research subject. Registries do entail prospective enrollment of participants, and thus requirements for ethical treatment of human subjects still apply, as in clinical trials (*see term:* Ethics and Privacy).

VALUE AND USE

Registry patients or participants are central to the purpose and success of these programs. Importantly, registry patient populations typically reflect real-world patient populations, with the variability in demographics, comorbidities, and treatment profiles normally seen in a specific condition, allowing the findings of these programs to often be more generalizable than traditional clinical trial findings.

ISSUES

Registry patients or participants are frequently and incorrectly referred to as subjects.

BIBLIOGRAPHY

46.102(f): Definition of human subject. Department of Health and Human Services. http://www.gpo.gov/fdsys/pkg/CFR-2011-title45-vol1/pdf/CFR-2011-title45-vol1-sec46-102.pdf. Accessed April 24, 2013.

Chapter 8. Principles of registry ethics, data ownership, and privacy. In: Gliklich RE, Dreyer NA, eds. *Registries for Evaluating Patient Outcomes: A User's Guide*. 2nd ed. (Prepared by Outcome DEcIDE Center [Outcome Sciences, Inc. d/b/a Outcome] under contract no. HHSA290200500351 T03.) AHRQ Publication No. 10-EHC049. Rockville, MD: Agency for Healthcare Research and Quality; 2010:167-204.

Research Questions

BRIEF DEFINITION

Questions of relevance to the scientific objectives.

EXPLANATION

The questions, which should be accurately and precisely defined, may either be related to clinical research or to clinical quality and outcomes. Clinical research (*see term:* Clinical Effectiveness and Comparative Effectiveness) is an attempt to derive generalizable new knowledge by addressing clearly defined questions using systematic and rigorous methods. Clinical quality and outcomes research are intended to inform the management of health care delivery services.

VALUE AND USE

Research questions in observational research are typically hypothesis generating or evidence building, rather than hypothesis testing, where a null hypothesis is defined *a priori* and statistical testing for significance is performed. The research question drives the conceptual framework of the study (*see term:* Statistical Inference and Hypothesis Testing).

BIBLIOGRAPHY

The Yeshiva Fatherhood Project. Introducing qualitative hypothesis-generating research. http://www.nyupress.org/webchapters/0814706940chapt1.pdf. Accessed April 24, 2013.

Chapter 2. Planning a registry. In: Gliklich RE, Dreyer NA, eds. *Registries for Evaluating Patient Outcomes: A User's Guide*. 2nd ed. (Prepared by Outcome DEcIDE Center [Outcome Sciences, Inc. d/b/a Outcome] under contract no. HHSA290200500351 T03.) AHRQ Publication No. 10-EHC049. Rockville, MD: Agency for Healthcare Research and Quality; 2010:23-52.

Vandenbroucke JP. Alvan Feinstein and the art of consulting: how to define a research question. *J Clin Epidemiol*. 2002;55:1176-1177.

Validity

BRIEF DEFINITION

The extent to which a concept, conclusion or measurement is well founded and corresponds accurately to the real world.

EXPLANATION

The validity of a measurement tool is considered to be the degree to which the tool measures what it claims to measure, and the trustworthiness of the conclusions of the study as they apply to the sample observed and the context used in the study (*see term:* Instrument or Scale Validation). Also refers to the extent to which study results overall are free from bias, and that the reported association between cause and effect (between exposure and outcome) is not due to unmeasured or uncontrolled-for variables.

VALUE AND USE

Validity is an essential characteristic of models and measurements used in outcomes research. If data are not accurately measured or not analyzed in models representing real systems, there is a significant risk of inaccurate or incomplete conclusions.

ISSUES

Observational research in general, including registries, is sometimes seen as being strong on external validity but weaker on internal validity, most notably when the observational research is drawing inference from comparisons between nonrandomized cohorts.

BIBLIOGRAPHY

Chapter 3. Registry design. In: Gliklich RE, Dreyer NA, eds. *Registries for Evaluating Patient Outcomes: A User's Guide*. 2nd ed. (Prepared by Outcome DEcIDE Center [Outcome Sciences, Inc. d/b/a Outcome] under contract no. HHSA290200500351 T03.) AHRQ Publication No. 10-EHC049. Rockville, MD: Agency for Healthcare Research and Quality; 2010:53-78.

American Educational Research Association, American Psychological Association, and National Research Council on Measurement in Education. *Standards for Educational and Psychological Testing*. Washington, DC: AERA; 1999.

Nunnally JC, Bernstein I. *Psychometric Theory*. 2nd ed. New York, NY: McGraw-Hill Book Company; 1978.

Cook DA, Beckman TJ. Current concepts in validity and reliability for psychometric instruments: theory and application. *Am J Med*. 2006;119:166.e7–166.e16.

Frost MH, Reeve BB, Liepa AM, et al. What is sufficient evidence for the reliability and validity of patient-reported outcome measures? *Value Health*. 2007;10:S94–S105.

Esposito D, ed. *Reliability and Validity of Data Sources for Outcomes Research & Disease and Health Management Programs*. Lawrenceville, NJ: ISPOR; 2013.

» *Internal Validity*

BRIEF DEFINITION

The extent to which the effects detected in a study are truly caused by the treatment or exposure in the study sample, rather than being due to other biasing effects of extraneous variables.

EXPLANATION

Internal validity occurs when a study design assures that only the variable being studied is able to affect the study's outcome and that all other variables have been identified, measured, and/or controlled.

VALUE AND USE

While ensuring study validity is more challenging in an observational study than in an RCT, current standards and design approaches in observational research provide important guidance in understanding and controlling for confounders, and in optimizing validity (*see term:* Analysis Techniques).

ISSUES

There are a number of threats to internal validity, which will vary among studies. For example, the history of the study may affect its validity, if events occurring between successive measurements impact the study's variables. Similarly, selection bias (*see term:* Selection Bias) may be a factor if different subgroups of patients are either selected or excluded from the registry. There are numerous other potential threats and confounders to a specific study, and the possible confounders will vary by the type of study, the study process/design, and the patient population being studied. Potential confounders should be explored in depth during the design phase of a registry, addressed in both the design and analytic approaches to the study, acknowledged in the publishing and reporting of results, and reflected in the strength of conclusions, as appropriate (*see term:* Confounders/Covariates).

BIBLIOGRAPHY

Fayers PM, Machin D. *Quality of Life: Assessment, Analysis, and Interpretation*. Chichester, UK: John Wiley & Sons Ltd; 2000.

Messick S. Validity. In: Linn RL, ed. *Educational Measurement*. 3rd ed. National Council on Measurement in Education and American Council on Education, Series in Higher Education. Phoenix, AZ: Oryx Press; 1993.

Messick S. Validity of psychological assessment: validation of inferences from person's responses and performances as scientific inquiry into score meaning. *Am Psychol*. 1995;50: 741-749.

Pedhazur EJ, Schmelkin LP. *Measurement, Design and Analysis: An Integrated Approach*. Hillsdale, NJ: Lawrence Erlbaum Associates; 1991.

Streiner DL, Norman GR. *Health Measurement Scales: A Practical Guide to Their Development and Use*. 2nd ed. New York, NY: Oxford University Press; 1995.

Chapter 3. Registry design. In: Gliklich RE, Dreyer NA, eds. *Registries for Evaluating Patient Outcomes: A User's Guide*. 2nd ed. (Prepared by Outcome DEcIDE Center [Outcome Sciences, Inc. d/b/a Outcome] under contract no. HHSA290200500351 T03.) AHRQ Publication No. 10-EHC049. Rockville, MD: Agency for Healthcare Research and Quality; 2010:53-78.

» *External Validity*

BRIEF DEFINITION

The extent to which the (internally valid) results of a study can be held to be true for other cases, (ie, different populations) or the extent to which the conclusions of the study can be generalized to populations and contexts other than those sampled and used in the study.

EXPLANATION

Often referred to as generalizability, the strong external validity of patient registries is achieved by the inclusion of a typical patient sample from a potentially heterogeneous patient population (*see term:* Patient Recruitment).

VALUE AND USE

Patient registries are generally designed to have strong external validity so that their population will be representative and relevant to decision makers.

ISSUES

As in internal validity, a number of factors may jeopardize external validity. These factors will vary among studies, but should be explored and addressed in-depth during a study's design phase. Some examples of threats or confounders to external validity include situational factors (eg, setting, timing, location), or pre-post test interaction (eg, when the findings are only observed when a pretest or post-test is administered). The generalizability of results should be highlighted in research reports, in particular noting any limitations to extending results to other patient populations and health care settings of interest.

BIBLIOGRAPHY

Fayers PM, Machin D. *Quality of Life: Assessment, Analysis, and Interpretation*. West Sussex, UK: John Wiley & Sons Ltd; 2000.

Messick S. Validity. In: Linn RL, ed. *Educational Measurement*. 3rd ed. National Council on Measurement in Education and American Council on Education, Series in Higher Education. Phoenix, AZ: Oryx; 1993.

Messick S. Validity of psychological assessment: validation of inferences from person's responses and performances as scientific inquiry into score meaning. *Am Psychol*. 1995;50:741-749.

Pedhazur EJ, Schmelkin LP. *Measurement, Design and Analysis: An Integrated Approach*. Hillsdale, Michigan: Erlbaum Associates Publishers; 1991.

Streiner DL, Norman GR. *Health Measurement Scales: A Practical Guide to Their Development and Use*. 2nd ed. New York, NY: Oxford University Press; 1995.

Chapter 3. Registry design. In: Gliklich RE, Dreyer NA, eds. *Registries for Evaluating Patient Outcomes: A User's Guide*. 2nd ed. (Prepared by Outcome DEcIDE Center [Outcome Sciences, Inc. d/b/a Outcome] under contract no. HHSA290200500351 T03.) AHRQ Publication No. 10-EHC049. Rockville, MD: Agency for Healthcare Research and Quality; 2010:53-78.

Study Limitations

BRIEF DEFINITION

Any weaknesses or shortcomings of the current study approach in terms of design, patient selection, data availability, and potential biases.

EXPLANATION

A full description of study limitations is an important aspect of all study reporting. Reporting of findings based on registry studies should also incorporate comparisons to other types of evidence (for instance, randomized controlled trials) and a discussion of potential reasons for any observed differences in findings.

VALUE AND USE

Appropriate reporting of limitations is essential for understanding research findings, areas and direction of potential biases, and the strength of the evidence compared to other studies. Describing limitations encountered in conducting a study may also help researchers better design future studies.

ISSUES

Identifying and discussing limitations is by nature a subjective process, and one that must be conducted *post hoc*. Discussion of limitations requires an overall appraisal of any problems with measurement, design, and internal/external validity. Authors are advised to describe any such issues in the context of the original rationale for the study, and reflect on new information gained (even if imperfect), as well as areas where the study findings may fall short of definitively answering the research question(s) (*see term:* Reporting and Dissemination of Registry-Based Studies).

BIBLIOGRAPHY

Ioannidis JP. Limitations are not properly acknowledged in the scientific literature. *J Clin Epidemiol*. 2007;60:324-329.

Transparency

BRIEF DEFINITION

A characteristic defined by the availability and clarity of key information on the rationale, methodology, and support (including funding) used to collect, analyze, and publish registry data.

EXPLANATION

Transparency in design of a registry can help to ensure that analyses and publications arising from registry data are properly evaluated with regard to validity and potential bias. Given the large number of individuals and organizations who may be involved with planning, implementing, and analyzing a registry, often over a long period of time, careful documentation will assist internal stakeholders as well as external audiences.

VALUE AND USE

Transparency in reporting facilitates interpretation of the study by other researchers as well as health care decision makers, and may lead to faster adoption of results.

ISSUES

Observational studies have received less attention than clinical trials in the quest for complete and timely reporting of study results. Postmarketing and registry studies play important roles in evidence development, however, and efforts to increase transparency should encompass these observational studies as well. Safety, comparative effectiveness, compliance and adherence, and variability among patient subgroups are all areas related to the translation of clinical trial results into routine practice settings. Full reporting of such studies, including negative results, is necessary for a complete picture of the evidence on medical interventions (*see terms:* Reporting Requirements; Reporting and Dissemination of Registry-Based Studies). Given the limitations on manuscript length in print journals and the frequent complexity of study design and analytic models in observational research, some authors have called for availability of the detailed protocol, coding definitions, and other methodologic detail on the journal's or researcher's website.

BIBLIOGRAPHY

Zarin DA, Tse T. Medicine. Moving toward transparency of clinical trials. *Science*. 2008;319: 1340-1342.

Andrews EB, Eaton S. Additional considerations in longitudinal database research. *Value Health*. 2003;6:85-87.

Reproducibility

BRIEF DEFINITION

Reproducibility refers to the ability of other investigators to re-create the findings of a study, if the study were to be repeated using the design of the original investigators.

EXPLANATION

Accurate and transparent reporting of all aspects of the study, such as study design, data collection, data analysis, etc., plays a critical role in reproducibility. Appropriate documentation of initial planning steps and decisions is needed for eventual dissemination of findings to the broader scientific community.

VALUE AND USE

Reproducibility is important for regulators, payers and other researchers to understand and build from the current research. Results which are able to be validated in independent datasets can lend credence to the findings, especially in the case of observational data.

ISSUES

The Methods section in published reports of observational studies can be limited. In one review, most articles failed to show sufficient or satisfactory quality of reproducibility, based on the descriptions in the Methods section. Methods sections of manuscripts or study reports should give thorough, transparent attention to all measures taken to minimize bias and should identify and justify all departures from the *a priori* analysis plan, if available (*see term:* Reporting and Dissemination of Registry-Based Studies).

BIBLIOGRAPHY

Patrick S, Hofer E, Lutz F. Evaluation of published clinical studies for reproducibility, comparability and adherence to evidence-based methods. *Am J Dent.* 2002;15:26-30.

Shao J, Chow SC. Reproducibility probability in clinical trials. *Stat Med.* 2002;21:1727-1742.

ISPOR Code of Ethics. International Society for Pharmacoeconomics and Outcomes Research. http://www.ispor.org/workpaper/CodeOfEthics.asp. Published March 2008. Accessed April 24, 2013.

Outcomes/End Points

Outcomes are the end results of a health care practice or intervention, and the effect of the health care process on the health and well-being of patients and populations. Outcomes provide evidence about the benefits, risks, and results of interventions. However, outcome measures are broader than just traditional biomedical (clinical) outcomes, such as morbidity and mortality. Outcomes or outcome end points include effects that people experience and care about, such as changes in the ability to function and quality of life. These outcomes, also known as PROs, are increasingly used in regulatory decisions. Health economic outcomes provide evidence on financial aspects of health care decisions, such as direct/indirect costs, burden of illness and cost-effectiveness. This outcome evidence allows for more informed decisions by clinicians, decision makers, payers and patients.

Outcomes/End Points

BRIEF DEFINITION

Prespecified outcomes measures that are related to the registry's key research question(s).

EXPLANATION

Before a clinical trial begins, researchers must determine what outcomes or end points they will monitor in order to be able to reach meaningful conclusions about the effect of the intervention they are studying. Unlike clinical trials, however, many registries do not refer to the variables they are observing or measuring as end points. Instead, key registry questions are defined at the registry's outset; these questions then drive the selection of outcomes measures that will be used to evaluate the questions.

VALUE AND USE

As in clinical trials, it is critical to identify up-front the key outcomes or measures to be studied in a registry. These outcomes may be revised throughout the program, but having prespecified objectives and outcomes to be measured is key to the study's scientific credibility and strength.

ISSUES

Registries are by definition more broad and adaptable than clinical trials. They do require, however, a strong study design that minimizes the likelihood of bias, loss-to-follow-up and missing data (*see terms:* Missing Observations; Strategies for Handling Missing Observations) and they do require analytic approaches that account for any bias and handle any missing observations, particularly for those outcome measures that are key to the registry's key research question(s).

BIBLIOGRAPHY

Chapter 2. Planning a registry. In: Gliklich RE, Dreyer NA, eds. *Registries for Evaluating Patient Outcomes: A User's Guide.* 2nd ed. (Prepared by Outcome DEcIDE Center [Outcome Sciences, Inc. d/b/a Outcome] under contract no. HHSA290200500351 T03.) AHRQ Publication No. 10-EHC049. Rockville, MD: Agency for Healthcare Research and Quality; 2010:23-52.

Dreyer NA, Schneeweiss S, McNeil BJ, et al. GRACE principles: recognizing high-quality observational studies of comparative effectiveness. *Am J Manag Care.* 2010;16:467-471.

Efficacy

» *Clinical Effectiveness*

BRIEF DEFINITION

The outcome of an intervention when it is administered under normal care circumstances to a general population, ie, real-world clinical care.

EXPLANATION

Clinical effectiveness studies evaluate patient outcomes where real-world conditions introduce multiple variables (including concomitant medications and co-morbidities) that potentially affect patient outcomes from a treatment regimen. Effectiveness should not be confused with efficacy, which refers to the rate of positive response or other patient outcomes in a controlled clinical trial setting where variation in response due to factors other than the intervention of interest is limited, to the extent this is possible. Effectiveness measures can involve intermediate outcomes (used as proxy measures for final outcomes or to predict an expected final outcome) or final clinical outcomes (lifetime or long-term beneficial or harmful outcome of an intervention in terms of morbidity and mortality), or may be designed to capture both.

VALUE AND USE

The measurement of clinical effectiveness in the real world better reflects the population exposed to the intervention, and is more generalizable (*see term:* External Validity).

ISSUES

Clinical effectiveness studies, including registries, have advantages for translation into clinical practice due to the broad population studied and the opportunity to assess long-term outcomes in a naturalistic setting. However, as observational studies, patient registries cannot minimize bias by random allocation to treatment groups and thus cannot establish causal relationships in the same manner as RCTs. Effectiveness studies, in the form of observational studies and patient registries, must therefore rely on other statistical methods to reduce bias in measuring treatment effects (*see terms:* Selection Bias; Risk-Adjustment Techniques). In addition, measures other than efficacy/effectiveness alone may also be relevant in evaluating the value of an intervention.

BIBLIOGRAPHY

Nasrallah HA, Smeltzer DJ. *Contemporary Diagnosis and Management of the Patient with Schizophrenia*. Newtown, PA: Handbooks in Health Care; 2002.

Olfson M. Emerging methods in mental health outcomes research. *J Pract Psychiatry Behav Health*. 1999;5:20-24.

Streiner DL. The 2 "Es" of research: efficacy and effectiveness trials. *Can J Psychiatry*. 2002;47:552-556.

Tandon R, Jibson MD. Efficacy of newer generation antipsychotics in the treatment of schizophrenia. *Psychoneuroendocrinology*. 2003;28:9-26.

Nasrallah HA, Targum SD, Tandon R, et al. Defining and measuring clinical effectiveness in the treatment of schizophrenia. *Psychiatr Serv*. 2005;56:273-282.

Kozma CM, Reeder CE, Schulz RM. Economic, clinical, and humanistic outcomes: a planning model for pharmacoeconomic research. *Clin Ther*. 1993;15:1121-1132.

» *Comparative Effectiveness*

BRIEF DEFINITION

The comparison of different interventions in a naturalistic setting rather than the more controlled setting of a clinical trial.

EXPLANATION

After efficacy of specific interventions has been established by RCTs, evidence gaps typically remain about how well patients will respond to the intervention outside of the narrow population generally eligible for trials. Trials performed for initial regulatory approval may be limited in comparators studied, follow-up duration, and subgroups identified, as well as patient population. Comparative effectiveness research differs from clinical efficacy as it attempts to systematically assess differences in real-world outcomes of available interventions.

VALUE AND USE

Observational studies, in general, and patient registries in particular, are potentially great sources for comparative effectiveness research.

ISSUES

Patient registries cannot minimize bias by random allocation to treatment groups, and thus, cannot establish causal relationships in the same manner as RCTs. Comparative effectiveness studies based on observational studies and patient registries, must therefore rely on statistical methods to reduce bias in measuring and comparing treatment effects (*see term:* Risk-Adjustment Techniques).

BIBLIOGRAPHY

Velentgas P, Dreyer NA, Nourjah P, et al. *Developing a Protocol for Observational Comparative Effectiveness Research: A User's Guide*. AHRQ Publication No. 12(13)-EHC099. Rockville, MD: Agency for Healthcare Research and Quality; 2013. www.effectivehealthcare.ahrq.gov/Methods-OCER.cfm. Accessed April 14, 2013.

Forrow S, Campion DM, Herrinton LJ, et al. The organizational structure and governing principles of the Food and Drug Administration's Mini-Sentinel pilot program. *Pharmacoepidemiol Drug Saf.* 2012;21:12-17.

Dreyer NA. Making observational studies count: shaping the future of comparative effectiveness research. *Epidemiology.* 2011;22:295-297.

Dreyer NA, Tunis S, Berger M, et al. Why observational studies should be among the tools used in comparative effectiveness research. *Health Aff.* 2010;29:1818-1825.

Dreyer NA, Schneeweiss S, McNeil BJ, et al. GRACE principles: recognizing high-quality observational studies of comparative effectiveness. *Am J Manag Care.* 2010;16:467-471.

Dreyer N. Generating evidence for decision making. *Am J Epidemiol.* 2010;171:S158-S165.

Dreyer NA, Rubino A, L'Italien GJ, Schneeweiss S. Developing good practice guidance for non randomized studies of comparative effectiveness: a workshop on quality and transparency. *Pharmacoepidemiol Drug Safety.* 2009;18:S123.

U.S. Department of Health & Human Services. Federal Coordinating Council for Comparative Effectiveness Research: Report to the President and the Congress. Published June 30, 2009. www.hhs.gov/recovery/programs/cer/cerannualrpt.pdf. Accessed April 24, 2013.

Sox HC, Helfand M, Grimshaw J, et al. Comparative effectiveness research: challenges for medical journals. *J Clin Epidemiol.* 2010;63:862-864.

Tunis SR, Benner J, McClellan M. Comparative effectiveness research: policy context, methods development and research infrastructure. *Stat Med.* 2010;29:1963-1976.

Schneeweiss S. Developments in post-marketing comparative effectiveness research. *Clin Pharmacol Ther.* 2007;82:143-156.

For further information on comparative effectiveness and economic evaluation, please see ISPOR Comparative Effectiveness Research Methods and Economic Evaluation Methods, Good Research Practice Reports at http://www.ispor.org/workpaper/practices_index.asp.

In addition, the following ISPOR good research practice reports may be helpful:

Berger ML, Dreyer N, Anderson F, et al. Prospective observational studies to assess comparative effectiveness: The ISPOR Good Research Practices Task Force Report. *Value Health*. 2012;15:217-230.

Hoaglin DC, Hawkins N, Jansen JP, et al. Conducting indirect-treatment-comparison and network meta-analysis studies: report of the ISPOR Task Force on Indirect Treatment Comparisons Good Research Practices: part 2. *Value Health*. 2011;14:429-437.

Jansen JP, Fleurence R, Devine B, et al. Interpreting indirect treatment comparisons and network meta-analysis for health-care decision making: report of the ISPOR Task Force on Indirect Treatment Comparisons Good Research Practices: part 1. *Value Health*. 2011;14:417-428.

Safety

Evaluation of treatment safety is increasingly critical, as regulators and payers today require some ongoing analysis of longer-term safety on virtually all new approved medications. Increasingly, registries are being developed as quality improvement initiatives with measures of safety included as markers of clinical quality of care. Specific types of safety measures, largely in the context of pharmaceutical products, are described below. It should be noted, however, that the measurement of patient safety is also critical to the evaluation of medical devices, procedures, or interventions.

» *Adverse Events*

BRIEF DEFINITION

Per International Conference on Harmonisation of Technical Requirements for Registration of Pharmaceuticals for Human Use (ICH) guidelines, an adverse event (AE) is any untoward medical occurrence in a patient or clinical-investigation subject administered a pharmaceutical product and which does not necessarily have a causal relationship with this treatment (*see term:* International Conference on Harmonization [ICH]: Good Clinical Practice [GCP]).

EXPLANATION

AEs may or may not be related to a product exposure; however, in the postmarketing setting, adverse drug reactions (ADRs) are a response to a drug which is noxious and unintended and which occurs at doses normally used for prophylaxis, diagnosis, or therapy of disease, or for modification of physiological function.

VALUE AND USE

Harmonized AE definitions and reporting requirements allow a systematic collection of safety-related information during clinical trials and observational studies (*see terms:* Reporting of Safety Outcomes; Reporting Requirements). Collection of AEs in patient registries can provide important information regarding a product's established safety profile, risks unknown at the time of product approval and product safety in patient populations not previously exposed to the product.

ISSUES

As sites participating in registries may not be accustomed to AE reporting to regulatory authorities, and the expectations for reporting, and for ensuring compliance with the regulations governing postmarketing AE reporting, these details must be clearly defined in the registry protocol (*see term:* Site Start-up).

BIBLIOGRAPHY

Edwards IR, Biriell C. Harmonisation in pharmacovigilance. *Drug Saf.* 1994;10:93-102.

European Medicines Agency. ICH Topic E2A. Clinical safety data management: definitions and standards for expedited reporting. 1995. http://www.emea.europa.eu/docs/en_GB/document_library/Scientific_guideline/2009/09/WC500002749.pdf. Published June 1995. Accessed April 24, 2013.

Fletcher AP. Spontaneous adverse drug reaction reporting vs. event monitoring: a comparison. *J R Soc Med.* 1991;84:341-344.

Mann R, Andrews E, eds. *Pharmacovigilance.* Chichester, UK: John Wiley & Sons; 2002.

Sills JM, Tanner LA, Milstien JB. Food and drug administration monitoring of adverse drug reactions. *Am J Hosp Phar.* 1986;43:2764-2770.

Talbot JC, Nilsson BS. Pharmacovigilance in the pharmaceutical industry. *Br J Clin Pharmacol.* 1998;45:427-431.

» *Passive Safety Surveillance*

BRIEF DEFINITION

The process of obtaining safety information through spontaneous reporting of AEs by physicians, patients and hospitals.

EXPLANATION

Passive safety surveillance generally refers to collection of AE data only as voluntary, unprompted reporting initiated by the patient or health care provider. This contrasts with active safety surveillance, in which there is a more structured and comprehensive collection of AEs (*see term:* Active Safety Surveillance).

VALUE AND USE

In patient registries where product safety is not an explicit objective, sites may be instructed to follow their normal practices for reporting spontaneous AEs directly to the relevant regulatory authorities, rather than to the registry itself.

ISSUES

Passive surveillance systems, such as the FDA's MedWatch program or the Vaccine Adverse Event Reporting System (VAERS), have been a cornerstone of pharmacovigilance but are inherently reactive and may lack sufficient detail to evaluate potential safety signals. The degree of underreporting is not known, but is assumed to be substantial.

BIBLIOGRAPHY

Ahmad SR, Freiman JP, Graham DJ, Nelson RC. Quality of adverse drug experience reports submitted by pharmacists and physicians to the FDA. *Pharmacoepidemiol Drug Saf.* 1996;5:1-7.

Rodriguez EM, Staffa JA, Graham DJ. The role of databases in drug postmarketing surveillance. *Pharmacoepidemiol Drug Saf.* 2001;10:407-410.

Varricchio F, Iskander J, Destefano F, et al. Understanding vaccine safety information from the Vaccine Adverse Event Reporting System. *Pediatr Infect Dis J.* 2004;23:287-294.

Vaccine Adverse Event Reporting System. http://vaers.hhs.gov/about/index. Updated April 12, 2013. Accessed April 24, 2013.

Harmark L, van Grootheest A. Pharmacovigilance: methods, recent developments and future perspectives. *Eur J Clin Pharmacol.* 2008;64:743-752.

» *Active Safety Surveillance*

BRIEF DEFINITION

The process of obtaining follow-up safety information from physicians or their patients that have received treatment. The patient is typically prompted by a set of specific questions regarding the tolerance of a product. Active surveillance may also include active use of signal-detection methods utilizing existing data sources, such as electronic medical records and administrative databases.

EXPLANATION

Active safety surveillance is emerging as an important complement to established passive-surveillance mechanisms.

VALUE AND USE

Active safety surveillance may be used as either a hypothesis-generating tool or a means of confirmation for existing hypotheses (*see term:* Statistical Inference and Hypothesis Testing). Patient registries may be used to generate safety data generally, or for specific AEs of interest, or to address safety issues in specific patient populations. The prospective nature of patient registries may allow for more detailed information regarding exposure, adherence/persistence, and covariates of interest that may not be found systematically in existing databases or records.

ISSUES

In order to conduct meaningful analyses, the study population must be well defined and appropriate epidemiologic methods should be applied to address critical components, including potential selection bias, sources of confounding and multiple comparisons (*see term:* Analysis Techniques; Selection Bias).

BIBLIOGRAPHY

Alghabban A. *Dictionary of Pharmacovigilance.* London: Pharmaceutical Press; 2004.

Dreyer NA, Sheth N, Trontell A, Gliklich RE. Good practices for handling adverse events detected through patient registries. *Drug Inf J.* 2008;42:421-428.

Lindquist M, Stahl M, Bate A, et al. A retrospective evaluation of a data mining approach to aid finding new adverse drug reaction signals in the WHO international database. *Drug Saf.* 2000;23:533-542.

O'Neill RT. Biostatistical considerations in pharmacovigilance and pharmacoepidemiology: linking quantitative risk assessment in pre-market licensure application safety data, post-market alert reports and formal epidemiological studies. *Stat Med.* 1998;17: 1851-1858.

U.S. Department of Health and Human Services. Food and Drug Administration. Center for Drug Evaluation and Research (CDER). Center for Biologics Evaluation and Research (CBER). Guidance for Industry: Good pharmacovigilance practice and pharmacoepidemiologic assessment. http://www.fda.gov/downloads/RegulatoryInformation/Guidances/UCM126834.pdf. Published March 2005. Accessed April 24, 2013.

» *Reporting of Safety Outcomes*

BRIEF DEFINITION

Safety reporting here refers to how AEs are defined, described and assessed in the publication and dissemination of registry results. (Note that the phrase "AE reporting" is also used to refer to reporting of events to regulatory authorities while the study is ongoing—this type of AE reporting is mentioned above) (*see terms:* Adverse Events; Reporting and Dissemination of Registry-Based Studies).

EXPLANATION

Components of safety reporting in publications may include incidence and type of event, characterizations of severity, the level of surveillance used (active/passive), coding systems used, and assessment of relationship to the intervention. It also can include whether specific events were asked about vs. open-ended questions regarding all events, and if all events are being reported or only the most frequent, most severe, or those of interest.

VALUE AND USE

For research studies with safety as a primary or secondary end point of interest, the details on the definition and assessment of the AEs are important to include in the methods of reports and publications. For economic studies based on registry data, AE occurrence will affect costs of care/cost-effectiveness. Therefore, appropriate reporting on AEs and the subsequent health care resource utilization are important.

ISSUES

In comparing rates of events with those observed in clinical trials or in other observational studies, care must be taken to assess differences between patient populations, comorbid diseases and concomitant medications, and the type of safety surveillance (active or passive) (*see terms:* Active Safety Surveillance; Passive Safety Surveillance).

BIBLIOGRAPHY

Berger ML, Bingefors K, Hedlom EC, et al, eds. *Healthcare Cost, Quality and Outcomes: ISPOR Book of Terms*. Lawrenceville, NJ: ISPOR; 2003.

Other Types of Outcomes

In addition to safety and clinical outcomes, a registry can also be used to collect information on outcomes that provide a broader assessment of the impact of a disease or clinical intervention. These include health-related quality of life (HRQOL), assessment of the costs associated with a disease and the cost-effectiveness of therapy (economic outcomes), levels of patient adherence and persistence to a care regimen and patient satisfaction with their treatment. In many cases, such outcomes are based on patient reports (referred to as patient-reported outcomes [PROs]). Registries can play a significant role in the assessment of these outcomes under real clinical practice conditions. These outcomes are described in more detail below.

» *Health-Related Quality of Life (HRQOL) Outcomes*

BRIEF DEFINITION

HRQOL refers to how the patient feels and functions, and extends beyond traditional measures of mortality and morbidity. It encompasses the domains of life directly affected by changes in health, including function, social activity, cognition, emotion, sleep and rest, energy and vitality, health perception, and general life satisfaction, and is measured by what the patient reports.

EXPLANATION

HRQOL emerged from research on health status. Measures were developed to identify common domains affected by disease that would allow clinicians to gauge the impact of a clinical condition. HRQOL can be assessed using generic instruments (eg, the 36-item Short Form Health Survey ie, [SF-36]) which can be used to measure quality of life (QOL) in any disease, or disease-specific instruments (eg, the Functional Assessment of Cancer Therapy-Prostate [FACT-P]) which are designed to capture elements associated with specific disease symptoms.

VALUE AND USE

While HRQOL can indicate treatment benefit and disease burden, it is a broad, multidimensional, theoretical construct used to organize, explain, and measure how a patient feels and functions overall in terms of specific health conditions or life in general *from the patient's perspective*. HRQOL typically targets health outcomes not fully appreciated by objective clinical measures or physician-reported outcomes (*see terms:* Instrument or Scale Validation; European Medicines Agency's (EMA) Guidance on HRQOL).

ISSUES

While there is great value in gathering data from the patient's self-assessment of the impacts of disease and treatment on their lives and well-being, HRQOL's data are subjective. However, there is a variety of scientific methods available to assess subjective outcomes (eg, utility measurement and psychometrics).

BIBLIOGRAPHY

Patrick DL, Erickson P. *Health Status and Health Policy; Quality of Life in Health Care Evaluation and Resource Allocation*. New York, NY: Oxford University Press; 1993.

Rogerson RJ. Environmental and health-related quality of life: conceptual and methodological similarities. *Soc Sci Med*. 1995;41:1373-1382.

Testa MA, Simonson DC. Assessment of quality-of-life outcomes. *N Eng J Med*. 1996;334: 835-840.

Albert SM, Teresi JA. Quality of life, definition and measurement. Encyclopedia of Aging. 2002. Encyclopedia.com. http://www.encyclopedia.com/doc/1G2-3402200344.html. Published 2002. Accessed April 24, 2013.

Berger ML, Bingefors K, Hedblom EC, et al. *Health Care Cost, Quality, and Outcomes: ISPOR Book of Terms*. Lawrenceville, NJ: ISPOR; 2003.

HTA 101: Glossary. National Information Center on Health Services Research and Health Care Technology (NICHSR). www.nlm.nih.gov/nichsr/hta101/ta101014.html. Updated August 16, 2012. Accessed April 24, 2013.

Acquadro C, Berzon R, Dubois D, et al. Incorporating the patient's perspective into drug development and communication: an ad hoc task force report of the Patient-Reported Outcomes (PRO) Harmonization Group meeting of the Food and Drug Administration, February 16, 2001. *Value Health*. 2003;6:522-531.

Leplege A, Hunt S. The problem of quality of life in medicine. *JAMA*. 1997;278:47-50.

Kennedy L, Craig AM. Global registries for measuring pharmacoeconomic and quality-of-life outcomes: focus on design and data collection, analysis and interpretation. *Pharmacoeconomics*. 2004;22:551-568.

For information on HRQOL and patient-reported outcomes, ISPOR has produced a number of PRO good research practice reports including the following below. They are available on the ISPOR Good Practices for Outcomes Research webpage at:: http://www.ispor.org/workpaper/practices_index.asp.

- Patient Reported Outcomes: Translation & cultural adaptation process
- Translation & linguistic validation of PRO instruments
- Content validity in existing PRO instruments & their modification
- Content validity in new PRO instruments Part 1 - Eliciting concepts for a new PRO Instrument
- Content validity in new PRO instruments Part 2 – Assessing respondent understanding ePRO: Changing mode of administration from paper to electronic

» *Direct Costs*

BRIEF DEFINITION

A cost that can be completely attributed to the production of a health care treatment; these costs are typically categorized as either direct medical or nonmedical costs. In health care, direct medical costs include those costs related to the specific delivery of health care, such as medications, doctor's visits, or medical equipment. Direct nonmedical costs are costs such as transportation to a hospital, or modifications to a home to allow for in-home care.

EXPLANATION

Direct costs include the cost of the resources whose consumption is wholly attributable to use of the health care intervention in question. These costs may include direct medical resource use, ie, hospitalization, physician, inpatient and outpatient costs, emergency department, nursing home care, hospice care, rehabilitation care, specialists' and other health professionals' care, the actual costs of interventions, diagnostic tests, prescription drugs, and medical supplies, and health care professional salaries, as well as direct nonmedical resource costs such as the cost of transporting patients.

VALUE AND USE

Understanding the true estimates of direct costs to treat a particular disease, whether on the patient or national level, allows for the prioritization of research funding among various diseases. Understanding the true estimates of direct costs among various alternatives of treatment allows for more informed decision making and ultimately for more efficient and impactful means of administering health care.

ISSUES

Any measurement of cost must be expressed in a context specific to the perspective: patient, provider, payer, society.

Hospital charges are often the only data available to calculate direct medical costs, particularly inpatient costs. Charges are typically higher than the actual costs to cover losses from patients who are unable to fully pay their expenses and procedures not covered by insurance companies, and to cover the costs of replacing and updating medical equipment.

Furthermore, most insurers negotiate reimbursement rates and receive substantial discounts off listed charges. Thus, hospital charges overestimate the underlying costs and do *not* accurately reflect actual costs. For more accurate cost estimates in the United States, the Centers for Medicare and Medicaid Services (CMS) can provide the cost-to-charge ratio for specific hospitals.

Finally, omission of nonmedical costs may provide an incomplete assessment of total direct health care costs associated with an intervention, if non-health care resources are consumed as part of the intervention or during follow-up. This may also bias cost-effectiveness analyses estimates that rely on such inputs, particularly when the perspective is that of the patient or society.

BIBLIOGRAPHY

Economic evaluation of public health preparedness and response efforts: cost analysis. Centers for Disease Control. http://www.cdc.gov/owcd/eet/Cost/fixed/3.html. Accessed April 24, 2013.

Drummond M, O'Brien B, Stoddart G, Torrance G. *Methods for the Economic Evaluation of Health Care Programmes*. New York, NY: Oxford University Press; 1997.

Gold MR, Siegel JE, Russell LB, Weinstein MC. *Cost-effectiveness in Health and Medicine*. New York, NY: Oxford University Press; 1996.

Weinstein MC, Siegel JE, Gold MR, et al. Recommendations of the panel on cost-effectiveness in health and medicine. *JAMA*. 1996;276:1253-1258.

Siegel JE, Weinstein MC, Russell LB, Gold MR. Recommendations for reporting cost-effectiveness analyses: panel on cost-effectiveness in health and medicine. *JAMA*. 1996;276:1339-1341.

Russell LB, Gold MR, Siegel JE, Daniels N, et al. The role of cost-effectiveness analysis in health and medicine: panel on cost-effectiveness in health and medicine. *JAMA*. 1996;276: 1172-1177.

Finkler SA. The distinction between costs and charges. *Ann Intern Med*. 1982;96:102-109.

Kennedy L, Craig AM. Global registries for measuring pharmacoeconomic and quality-of-life outcomes: focus on design and data collection, analysis and interpretation. *Pharmacoeconomics*. 2004;22:551-568.

» *Indirect Costs*

BRIEF DEFINITION

In health care, indirect costs are costs resulting from productivity losses, such as time lost from work (absenteeism) or reduced productivity at work (presenteeism) caused by the health problem or disease.

EXPLANATION

Indirect health care costs typically refer to the costs related to lost or reduced productivity because of illness, recruitment and training of replacement personnel for employees who can no longer work because of illness, and paid or unpaid employee's morbidity or mortality. Indirect costs are typically estimated using gross earnings lost.

VALUE AND USE

Indirect costs are important measures of the true, overall impact of a disease, and of its treatment.

ISSUES

Any measurement of cost must be expressed in a context specific to the perspective: patient, provider, payer, society.

Controversy exists about whether or not indirect costs and benefits should be included in economic evaluations of health services and programs. In addition, if they are included, there is also debate about how they should be measured. The inclusion of indirect costs and benefits is likely to advantage some groups and disadvantage others. The inclusion of indirect costs and benefits without constraints can result in *de facto* discrimination due to income disparities between genders and race or ethnic groups.

BIBLIOGRAPHY

Koopmanschap MA, Rutten FF. A practical guide for calculating indirect costs for disease. *Pharmacoeconomics*. 1996;10:460-466.

McKie J, Richardson J. Neglected Equity Issues in Cost Effectiveness Analysis—Part 2: Direct and Indirect Costs, the Preservation of Hope, the Rule of Rescue, Patient Adaptation, and the Ex Ante/Ex Post Distinction. Centre for Health Economics Research Papers 8/05. Melbourne, AU: Monash University Centre for Health Economics; 2005.

Health Economics Information Resources: A Self-Study Course. National Information Center on Health Services Research and Health Care Technology (NICHSR). http://www.nlm.nih.gov/nichsr/edu/healthecon/glossary.html. Updated April 22, 2013. Accessed April 24, 2013.

» *Cost-Effectiveness and Cost Utility*

BRIEF DEFINITION

Two types of economic analytical methods used to relate outcomes and costs of health care interventions.

EXPLANATION

A cost-effectiveness ratio is the difference in cost divided by the difference in effectiveness (eg, in survival, progression-free survival, or other defined response rate) associated with treatment alternatives. More specifically, the incremental cost-effectiveness ratio (ICER), the ratio between the increase in cost and the increase in mean effectiveness, is commonly used to compare interventions. Cost-utility analysis, unlike simple cost-effectiveness, allows comparisons across multiple interventions and can incorporate multiple outcomes using a quality-adjusted life year (QALY) as the measure of effectiveness, where the outcomes are adjusted by health state preference scores or utility weights

VALUE AND USE

Patient registries can provide important support for health economic analyses by supplying outcomes data (and standardized health state ratings such as the EQ-5D) for patient populations, including subgroups not previously studied, or over longer periods of time. The cost-effectiveness/cost-utility analysis is used as a tool to help stakeholders and/or policy makers in value-based decision making to allocate health resources more effectively. From a coverage perspective, payment determinations can therefore be informed by registries.

ISSUES

Cost-utility analyses (and QALYs) allow a common currency for purposes of resource allocation decisions, but have important limitations, specifically in the application to chronic diseases, preventative measures, psychiatric and emotional health outcomes, and conditions which significantly affect caregivers as well as patients. In addition, the appropriateness of specific monetary thresholds, a reflection of society's willingness to pay per QALY, is hotly debated, particularly in regards to medications for rare diseases or end-of-life support.

BIBLIOGRAPHY

Drummond M, O'Brien B, Stoddart G, Torrance G. *Methods for the Economic Evaluation of Health Care Programmes*. New York, NY: Oxford University Press; 1997.

Gold M, Siegel J, Russell L, Weinstein M, eds. *Cost-effectiveness in Health and Medicine*. New York, NY: Oxford University Press; 1996.

Koopmanschap M, Rutten F. A practical guide for calculating indirect costs for disease. *Pharmacoeconomics*. 1996;10:460-466.

Hunink M, Glasziou P, Siegel J, et al. *Decision-making in Health and Medicine: Integrating Evidence and Values*. Cambridge, UK: Cambridge University Press; 2001.

Weinstein M, Stason W. Foundations of cost-effectiveness analysis for health and medical practices. *N Engl J Med*. 1977;296:716-721.

Ramsey S, Willke R, Briggs A, et al. Good research practices for cost-effectiveness analysis alongside clinical trials: the ISPOR RCT-CEA Task Force report. *Value Health*. 2005;8: 521-533.

Hay JW, Smeeding J, Carroll NV, et al. Good research practices for measuring drug costs in cost effectiveness analyses: issues and recommendations: the ISPOR Drug Cost Task Force report—Part I. *Value Health*. 2010;13:3-7.

Garrison LP Jr, Mansley EC, Abbott TA III, et al. Good research practices for measuring drug costs in cost-effectiveness analyses: A societal perspective: the ISPOR Drug Cost Task Force report—Part II. *Value Health*. 2010;13:8-13.

Mansley EC, Carroll NV, Chen KS, et al. Good research practices for measuring drug costs in cost-effectiveness analyses: a managed care perspective: the ISPOR Drug Cost Task Force Report—Part III. *Value Health*. 2010;13:14-17.

Mullins CD, Seal B, Seoane-Vazquez E, et al. Good research practices for measuring drug costs in cost-effectiveness analyses: Medicare, Medicaid and other US government payers perspectives: the ISPOR Drug Cost Task Force report—Part IV. *Value Health*. 2010;13:18-24.

Mycka JM, Dellamano R, Kolassa EM, et al. Good research practices for measuring drug costs in cost effectiveness analyses: an industry perspective: the ISPOR Drug Cost Task Force report—Part V. *Value Health*. 2010;13:25-27.

Shi L, Hodges M, Drummond M, et al. Good research practices for measuring drug costs in cost-effectiveness analyses: an international perspective: the ISPOR Drug Cost Task Force report—Part VI. *Value Health*. 2010;13:28-33.

» *Compliance/Adherence*

BRIEF DEFINITION

Patient adherence to a care regimen prescribed by a physician or other health care provider, such as taking medications correctly, at the required frequency and dose and on time. (Note: Compliance and adherence are often used interchangeably, though in recent years the term adherence has been preferred as more patient-centric.)

EXPLANATION

Adherence encompasses a patient's active participation in his or her own health care including seeking medical advice, keeping appointments, following recommendations concerning lifestyle, as well as following medical regimens. Adherence is dependent on several factors that represent the burden of treatment. Treatment burden includes side effects and complexity of treatment; an example of the latter is a medication that should be taken with food. Adherence includes the patient's willingness and readiness to follow the prescribed dosing instructions. Noncompliance with medication may include failure to take medications, taking too much medication, taking a drug for the wrong reason, improper timing of drug administration or not having the prescription filled or refilled.

VALUE AND USE

Often nonadherence or inadequate adherence is a factor in reducing clinical effectiveness levels, particularly in the treatment of silent chronic diseases such as hypertension. It can also result in higher costs and/or waste of resources.

ISSUES

Measuring compliance/adherence levels presents practical challenges in both the clinical trial and registry settings. Factoring in *actual* compliance and persistence (*see term:* Persistence) is central to an accurate assessment of effectiveness and cost-effectiveness of therapy. However, a number of methodologies are now available for quantifying compliance/adherence, including electronic medication monitors and self-reported patient diaries. These methods can be used to compare the degree of compliance/adherence with different medications and to characterize factors that impact patient ability to comply with their overall treatment regimen.

BIBLIOGRAPHY

Cramer JA, Roy A, Burrell A, et al. Medication compliance and persistence: terminology and definitions. *Value Health*. 2008;11:44-47.

Cramer JA. Microelectronic systems for monitoring and enhancing patient compliance with medication regimens. *Drugs*. 1995;49:321-327.

Cramer JA, Spilker B, eds. *Patient Compliance in Medical Practice and Clinical Trials*. New York, NY: Raven Press; 1991.

Sullivan SD, Kreling DH, Hazlet TH. Non-compliance with medication regimens and subsequent hospitalization: a literature analysis and cost of hospitalization estimate. *J Res Pharm Econ*. 1990;2:19-33.

Urquhart J. Pharmacoeconomic consequences of variable patient compliance with prescribed drug regimens. *Pharmacoeconomics*. 1999;15:217-228.

Peterson AM, Nau DP, Cramer JA, et al. A checklist for medication compliance and persistence studies using retrospective databases. *Value Health*. 2007;10:3-12.

Hughes D, Cowell W, Koncz T, et al. Methods for integrating medication compliance and persistence in pharmacoeconomic evaluations. *Value Health*. 2007;10:498-509.

» *Persistence*

BRIEF DEFINITION

The duration of time from initiation of therapy to the patient effectively discontinuing therapy.

EXPLANATION

Persistence specifically refers to the time that the medication *is taken as prescribed* from the time of initiation to discontinuation.

VALUE AND USE

As with adherence and compliance, real-world observational studies and registries are the best design through which to assess treatment persistence (*see term:* Compliance/Adherence).

ISSUES

When there is variation in the prescribed dosing regimen, medications have situation-specific alterations in benefit/risk ratios, either due to increased risks or reduced benefits, or both. Inadequate compliance and nonpersistence with prescribed medication regimens result in increased morbidity and mortality from a wide variety of illnesses, as well as increased health care costs. Registries provide an ideal way to assess the impact of persistence patterns on health and economic outcomes in real clinical practice.

BIBLIOGRAPHY

Cramer JA. Microelectronic systems for monitoring and enhancing patient compliance with medication regimens. *Drugs.* 1995;49:321-327.

Cramer JA, Spilker B, eds. *Patient Compliance in Medical Practice and Clinical Trials.* New York, NY: Raven Press; 1991.

Sullivan SD, Kreling DH, Hazlet TH. Non-compliance with medication regimens and subsequent hospitalization: a literature analysis and cost of hospitalization estimate. *J Res Pharm Econ.* 1990;2:19-33.

Urquhart J. Pharmacoeconomic consequences of variable patient compliance with prescribed drug regimens. *Pharmacoeconomics.* 1999;15:217-228.

Cramer JA, Roy A, Burrell A, et al. Medication compliance and persistence: terminology and definitions. *Value Health.* 2008;11:44-47.

Peterson AM, Nau DP, Cramer JA, et al. A checklist for medication compliance and persistence studies using retrospective databases. *Value Health.* 2007;10:3-12.

Hughes D, Cowell W, Koncz T, et al. Methods for integrating medication compliance and persistence in pharmacoeconomic evaluations. *Value Health.* 2007;10:498-509.

» *Treatment Satisfaction*

BRIEF DEFINITION

A patient-reported outcome (PRO) measure defined as a patient's rating of his or her experience with the process and outcomes of treatment.

EXPLANATION

Treatment satisfaction is a relatively new PRO that was previously ignored or assumed in clinical practice. This concept is related to patients' views on their treatment. It is an important concept because it has implications to patient adherence and persistence with treatment. Treatment satisfaction represents an interaction of effectiveness, side effects and convenience of treatment domains within the scales of expectations, experiences and overall satisfaction among patients. Moreover, it has been shown to impact patient's intention to continue medication. Treatment Satisfaction Questionnaire for Medication (TSQM) (http://www.quintiles.com/tsqm) and the Diabetes Treatment Satisfaction Questionnaire (DTSQ) (http://www.musc.edu/dfm/RCMAR/DTSQ.html) are examples of tools measuring treatment satisfaction. The TSQM is a generic measure of treatment satisfaction with medication and has been validated for psychometric properties and linguistic transliteration. The domains of this tool include: effectiveness, side effects, convenience and global satisfaction. The DTSQ is a disease-specific tool for diabetes with domains related to hyper- and hypoglycemia and general health.

VALUE AND USE

Treatment satisfaction is often a factor that predicts adherence and persistence with treatment and hence, can have a large impact on outcomes. Access to measures of patients' satisfaction with several treatments also provides a point of comparison when considering different treatment options (for example: once a day dosing versus multiple dosing; single versus combination regimens, minimally invasive laparoscopic surgery versus invasive surgery). Information on treatment satisfaction can thus help: 1. patients and clinicians decide between the treatments; 2. identify aspects of interventions or regimens that need to be adapted; 3. identify and work with patients for whom the treatment may be challenging; 4. be another point of comparison along with other PROs for industry to provide a competitive advantage on their product(s).

ISSUES

Treatment satisfaction focuses on one aspect of satisfaction with medical care and involves the interaction of expectations, experiences, and satisfaction with medical treatment. There are proposed relationships with HRQOL and other preference-based measures. However there are very few validated tools to measure this concept (*see term:* Instrument or Scale Validation). Comparing treatment satisfaction between cohorts in a registry must keep in mind that different patients bring different expectations when undergoing treatments. For example, a rheumatoid arthritis patient initiating biologic therapy for the first time may have higher expectations of treatment effectiveness (and therefore satisfaction) than a similar patient initiating a new biologic therapy after having failed on 2 previous therapies.

BIBLIOGRAPHY

Atkinson MJ, Kumar R, Cappelleri JC, Hass SL. Hierarchical construct validity of the treatment satisfaction questionnaire for medication (TSQM version II) among outpatient pharmacy consumers. *Value Health.* 2005;8:S9-S24.

Atkinson MJ, Sinha A, Hass SL, et al. Validation of a general measure of treatment satisfaction, the Treatment Satisfaction Questionnaire for Medication (TSQM), using a national panel study of chronic disease. *Health Qual Life Outcomes.* 2004;2:12.

Bharmal M, Payne K, Atkinson MJ, et al. Validation of an abbreviated Treatment Satisfaction Questionnaire for Medication (TSQM-9) among patients on antihypertensive medications. *Health Qual Life Outcomes.* 2009;7:36.

Bradley C. Diabetes treatment satisfaction questionnaire. In: Bradley C, ed. *Handbook of Psychology and Diabetes.* Chur, Switzerland: Harwood Academic Publishers; 1994.

Kravitz RL. Patients' expectations for medical care: an expanded formulation based on review of the literature. *Med Care Res Rev.* 1996;53:3–27.

Kumar RN, Kirking DM, Hass SL, et al. The association of consumer expectations, experiences and satisfaction with newly prescribed medications. *Qual Life Res.* 2007;16:1127–1136.

Asadi-Lari M, Tamburini M, Gray D. Patients' needs, satisfaction, and health related quality of life: towards a comprehensive model. *Health Qual Life Outcomes.* 2004;2:32.

Peyrot M, Rubin RR. How does treatment satisfaction work? Modeling determinants of treatment satisfaction and preference. *Diabetes Care.* 2009;32:1411-1417.

Revicki DA. Patient assessment of treatment satisfaction: methods and practical issues. *Gut.* 2004;53:iv40-iv44.

Law A, Bounthavong M. Patient satisfaction and health and disease management. In: Esposito D, ed. *Reliability and Validity of Data Sources for Outcomes Research & Disease and Health Management Programs.* Lawrenceville, NJ: ISPOR; 2013.

General Study Design

Retrospective

BRIEF DEFINITION

The defining feature of a study that involves analysis of previously captured data. Collection of data on clinical end points, treatments, and related measures is recorded before commencement of the study.

EXPLANATION

Retrospective database studies can examine the health care utilization of patients in real-world settings. They can focus on economic and/or clinical outcomes and can be conducted from a variety of perspectives including those of patients, health care providers, payers, and society. In fact, a defining characteristic of retrospective studies is that they involve the analysis of data that has already been collected—usually for some purpose other than the study at hand.

VALUE AND USE

Patient registries are, by definition, assembled prospectively, but data on exposure, treatments and events occurring before enrollment may be assembled retrospectively at baseline. Retrospective databases are often very large (sometimes containing information on millions of individuals) and, because the information has already been collected, retrospective studies can be carried out more rapidly than clinical trials or prospective observational studies.

ISSUES

Observational studies, both retrospective and prospective, can be valuable because they provide information about health care treatments in real-world settings. Lack of randomization in these studies may result in unequal distribution of measured and unmeasured confounders across exposure groups that must be addressed in analyses (*see term:* Analysis Techniques).

BIBLIOGRAPHY

Anderson C. Measuring what works in health care. *Science*. 1994;263:1082.

Arnold R, Kotsanos J. Panel 3: Methodological issues in conducting pharmacoeconomic evaluations—retrospective and claims database studies. *Value Health*. 1999;2:82-87.

Garnick DW, Hendricks AM, Comstock CB. Measuring quality of care: fundamental information from administrative datasets. *Int J Qual Health Care*. 1994;6:163-177.

McGlynn EA, Damberg CL, Kerr EA, Brook RH. *Health Information Systems: Design Issues and Analytic Applications*. Santa Monica, CA: Rand Health; 1998.

Motheral B, Brooks J, Clark MA, et al. A checklist for retroactive database studies: report of the ISPOR Task Force on Retrospective Databases. *Value Health*. 2003;6:90-97.

Berger ML, Mamdani M, Atkins D, Johnson ML. Good research practices for comparative effectiveness research: defining, reporting and interpreting nonrandomized studies of treatment effects using secondary data sources: the ISPOR good research practices for retrospective database analysis task force report—Part I. *Value Health*. 2009;12:1044-1052.

Cox E, Martin BC, Van Staa T, et al. Good research practices for comparative effectiveness research: approaches to mitigate bias and confounding in the design of non-randomized studies of treatment effects using secondary data sources: the ISPOR good research practices for retrospective database analysis task force–Part II. *Value Health*. 2009;12:1053-1061.

Peterson AM, Nau DP, Cramer JA, et al. A checklist for medication compliance and persistence studies using retrospective databases. *Value Health*. 2007;10:3-12.

For information on observational study methods, please see the ISPOR Good Practices for Outcomes Research webpage at http://www.ispor.org/workpaper/practices_index.asp.

For information on how to assess and interpret observational studies, please see the ISPOR web-based questionnaire on assessing evidence in observational research studies at www.ispor.org.

Case-Control Study

BRIEF DEFINITION

A retrospective study in which past exposure of a group with an outcome is compared to the exposure of a group *without* the outcome.

EXPLANATION

A retrospective study model applied to registry data when the need is to determine what proportion of persons, with or without a certain outcome, has or had an exposure or characteristic of interest. In a case-control study, two groups are assembled: a group, or cases, with a given health outcome (eg, disease, AE) and; a group, or controls, without the outcome but otherwise considered comparable. Case-control studies involve a retrospective comparison between the 2 study groups to identify any possible causal exposures. Nesting a case-control study within a larger cohort study ensures that cases and controls are selected from the same population.

VALUE AND USE

Case-control studies are ideal for studying the etiology of rare diseases or health outcomes as significantly fewer subjects are needed than for a cohort study assessing the same outcomes. Case-control studies can be a more efficient way of studying an outcome of interest than cohort studies as they do not require the time and expense of following patients over time to observe the outcome (*see term:* Cohort Study). This type of study is particularly useful in situations where there is a long time lapse between the exposure of interest and the disease outcome.

ISSUES

Relative risk cannot be calculated directly from a case-control study as the incidence of disease cannot be estimated. The odds ratio is calculated instead, which roughly approximates the relative risk when the outcome is rare. Case-control studies may be impacted by problems with recall bias and difficulty in establishing a causal relationship, as the exposure is measured after the development of disease.

BIBLIOGRAPHY

Strom BL. Study designs available for pharmacoepidemiology studies. In: Strom BL, ed. *Pharmacoepidemiology*. 4th ed. Chichester, UK: John Wiley; 2005:17-26.

Chapter 3. Registry design. In: Gliklich RE, Dreyer NA, eds. *Registries for Evaluating Patient Outcomes: A User's Guide*. 2nd ed. (Prepared by Outcome DEcIDE Center [Outcome Sciences, Inc. d/b/a Outcome] under contract no. HHSA290200500351 T03.) AHRQ Publication No. 10-EHC049. Rockville, MD: Agency for Healthcare Research and Quality; 2010:53-78.

Meirik O. Cohort and case-control studies. In: Campana A, Dreifuss JJ, Sizonenko P, eds. *Reproductive Health*. Rome, Italy: Ares Serono Symposia Publications; 1993. http://www.gfmer.ch/Books/Reproductive_health/Cohort_and_case_control_studies.html. Accessed April 24, 2013.

Prospective

BRIEF DEFINITION

The defining feature of a study that involves analysis of prospectively captured data. Collection of data on clinical end points, treatments, and related measures is predefined in a study protocol before commencement of the study

» *Interventional*

Prospective interventional studies are those in which a prespecified protocol dictates that the provider administers some element of treatment (eg, a surgical procedure), drug therapy (including placebo), or use of a medical device (including sham or diagnostic tests) that may not necessarily be consistent with usual or real-world patient care. Patients may be randomized to treatment groups, as in an RCT.

EXPLANATION

Interventional studies, especially RCTs, are often used in hypothesis testing (*see term:* Statistical Inference and Hypothesis Testing). By definition, patient registries are not interventional.

» *Noninterventional/Observational*

A study design that observes the outcomes of treatment initiated through standard medical management, and does not dictate or mandate care. Care is typically not a result of randomization or other forms of patient assignment.

EXPLANATION

Synonymous with a naturalistic study; by definition, all patient registries are observational in design.

VALUE AND USE

Patient registries use observational study methods to collect uniform data in a specific population. Observational studies may be warranted when controlled experiments would be unethical or infeasible, or when the research question requires information regarding exposures and outcomes as they occur in routine clinical practice. Well-designed observational studies can provide important evidence that cannot be derived from the RCT setting, with strong internal and external validity (*see term:* Validity).

ISSUES

Regulations and guidelines are inconsistent internationally regarding the definitions of observational and interventional studies. Depending on local regulations, for example, blood tests and patient questionnaires may be considered interventional in some countries, particularly in Europe, but not in others. This distinction has implications for the regulations under which studies must be conducted, for the degree of health authority review and approval that is required, and for reporting requirements (*see terms:* Evaluating and Ensuring Registry Quality; Good Research Practice Considerations; Reporting Requirements).

In addition, due to the absence of randomization or other control of exposure, there is a potential for bias in observational studies which must be considered in the design and analysis. Observational studies may also be biased by what is known as the Hawthorne effect, when the behavior of patients (or participating investigators) may be influenced simply in response to being studied. This can be a particular problem when the study objectives include subjective outcomes such as treatment patterns, use or nonuse of diagnostic testing, and other outcomes dependent on individual clinical decisions, as well as patient outcomes such as adherence, or HRQOL.

In 2007, the Strengthening the Reporting of Observational Studies in Epidemiology (STROBE) statement was issued, which called for observational studies to conform to 22 criteria that would make their conclusions easier to understand and generalize (*see term:* STROBE).

BIBLIOGRAPHY

European Group for Blood and Marrow Transplantation. Guidelines for the conduct of registry based studies using the EBMT database. http://www.docstoc.com/docs/88206743/GUIDELINES-FOR-RETROSPECTIVE-STUDIES-USING-THE-EBMTREGISTRIES-v-1. Updated April 26, 2011. Accessed April 24, 2013.

Chapter 3. Registry design. In: Gliklich RE, Dreyer NA, eds. *Registries for Evaluating Patient Outcomes: A User's Guide*. 2nd ed. (Prepared by Outcome DEcIDE Center [Outcome Sciences, Inc. d/b/a Outcome] under contract no. HHSA290200500351 T03.) AHRQ Publication No. 10-EHC049. Rockville, MD: Agency for Healthcare Research and Quality; 2010:53-78.

von Elm E, Altman DG, Egger M, et al. The Strengthening the Reporting of Observational Studies in Epidemiology (STROBE) statement: guidelines for reporting observational studies. *PLoS Med*. 2007;4:e296.

Dreyer NA, Tunis SR, Berger M, et al. Why observational studies should be among the tools used in comparative effectiveness research. *Health Aff*. 2010;29:1818-1825.

Berger ML, Dreyer N, Anderson F, et al. Prospective observational studies to assess comparative effectiveness: the ISPOR Good Research Practices Task Force report. *Value Health*. 2012;15:217-230.

For information on how to assess and interpret prospective observational studies, please see the ISPOR web-based questionnaire on assessing evidence in observational research studies at www.ispor.org.

Cohort Study

BRIEF DEFINITION

A prospective, descriptive study model, applied in registries and for studies evaluating comparative effectiveness, safety, and/or quality of care. Cohort studies follow a group of persons with certain shared characteristics to observe whether or not they develop a particular end point or outcome over time.

EXPLANATION

Cohort studies may include patients with specific exposures (eg, to a specific drug or class of drugs) or disease of interest. Cohort studies may also include one or more comparison groups, in which data are collected concurrently using the same methods. Cohort studies may follow a population over a relatively short period of time (eg, six months) or even decades (eg, Nurses' Health Study). Cohort studies can also be conducted retrospectively using existing data sources.

VALUE AND USE

Both incidence rate and relative risk can be calculated in a cohort study. Cohort studies are particularly useful for studying rare exposures, as exposed patients are selectively enrolled in the study. Since cohort studies follow patients over time, the temporal relationship between exposure and disease can be clearly documented and detailed information about the exposure and outcomes can be collected in a controlled manner. Cohort studies are also useful because they allow the study of multiple outcomes for a particular exposure.

ISSUES

Cohort studies are not efficient for studying relatively rare diseases/outcomes. They can also be expensive and time consuming to conduct in comparison with other observational study designs.

BIBLIOGRAPHY

Strom BL. Study designs available for pharmacoepidemiology studies. In: Strom BL, ed. *Pharmacoepidemiology*. 4th ed. Chichester, UK: John Wiley & Sons; 2005:17-26.

Chapter 3. Registry design. In: Gliklich RE, Dreyer NA, eds. *Registries for Evaluating Patient Outcomes: A User's Guide*. 2nd ed. (Prepared by Outcome DEcIDE Center [Outcome Sciences, Inc. d/b/a Outcome] under contract no. HHSA290200500351 T03.) AHRQ Publication No. 10-EHC049. Rockville, MD: Agency for Healthcare Research and Quality; 2010:53-78.

Meirik O. Cohort and case-control studies. In: Campana A, Dreifuss JJ, Sizonenko P, eds. *Reproductive Health*. Rome, Italy: Ares Serono Symposia Publications; 1993. http://www.gfmer.ch/Books/Reproductive_health/Cohort_and_case_control_studies.html. Accessed April 24, 2013.

Usual Care

BRIEF DEFINITION

Health care delivery as it is exercised by the average professional in a particular health care environment.

EXPLANATION

Usual care, sometimes referred to as real-world care, can be assessed through an observational or noninterventional study. Patients are observed without undue interference by protocol demands.

VALUE AND USE

Usual care, or real-world care, is the desired context for patient registries.

ISSUES

Although usual care may be standardized around high-level evidence, and thus represent best current therapy (eg, aspirin therapy for acute coronary syndromes), it may also be highly variable and include both prudent and undesirable practices (*see term:* Standard of Care).

BIBLIOGRAPHY

Kennedy L, Craig A. Global registries for measuring pharmacoeconomic and quality of life outcomes: focus on design and data collection, analysis and interpretation. *Pharmacoeconomics*. 2004;22:551-568.

Thompson BT, Schoenfeld D. Usual care as the control group in clinical trials of nonpharmacologic interventions. *Proc Am Thorac Soc*. 2007;4:577-582.

The Seventh Report of the Joint National Committee on Prevention, Detection, and Treatment of High Blood Pressure. US Department of Health and Human Service. http://www.nhlbi.nih.gov/guidelines/hypertension/jnc7full.pdf. Published August 2004. Accessed April 24, 2013.

Standard of Care

BRIEF DEFINITION

A diagnostic and treatment process that a clinician should follow for a certain type of patient, illness, or clinical circumstance. In legal terms, it is the level at which the average prudent provider in a given community would practice. It is how similarly qualified practitioners would have managed the patient's care under the same or similar circumstances.

EXPLANATION

Standard of care, in the context of a registry, encompasses all typical treatment regimens and approaches that are commonly used to treat a particular condition.

VALUE AND USE

Standard of care is often designated as a comparator arm in a registry.

ISSUES

The standard of care can vary substantially by region or country which is important to consider in analytic design and interpretation of results.

BIBLIOGRAPHY

Annas GJ. *Standard of Care: The Law of American Bioethics*. New York, NY: Oxford University Press; 1993.

Definition of standard of care. MedicineNet.com. http://www.medterms.com/script/main/art.asp?articlekey=33263. Updated June 14, 2012. Accessed April 24, 2013.

Treatment Guidelines/Consensus

BRIEF DEFINITION

Guidelines or treatment algorithm for a specific therapy or disease.

EXPLANATION

Since a registry is observational in design, treatment guidelines are not mandated. Instead the registry is a reflection of how treatment guidelines are used in real clinical practice.

VALUE AND USE

Since treatment approaches are not mandated in a patient registry, specific treatment guidelines may be listed as a resource and reference for participating clinicians, but following those guidelines would not be required. A possible objective of a patient registry could, however, be to observe concordance with treatment guidelines, or the degree to which treatment guidelines are in fact followed.

ISSUES

Not all treatment guidelines or protocols are evidence based.

BIBLIOGRAPHY

Eden J, Wheatley B, McNeil B, Sox H. Developing trusted clinical practice guidelines. In: Eden J, Wheatley B, McNeil B, Sox H, eds. *Knowing What Works in Health Care: A Roadmap for the Nation*. Washington DC: The National Academies Press; 2008. http://www.nap.edu/openbook.php?record_id=12038&page=121. Accessed April 24, 2013.

National Guideline Clearinghouse. Agency for Healthcare Research and Quality. http://www.guideline.gov/. Updated April 22, 2013. Accessed April 24, 2013.

American College of Cardiology/American Heart Association (ACC/AHA) Joint Guidelines. http://my.americanheart.org/professional/StatementsGuidelines/ACCAHA-JointGuidelines_UCM_321694_Article.jsp. Accessed May 1, 2013.

Stakeholders

Primary Stakeholder

BRIEF DEFINITION

Those individuals/organizations responsible for creating and funding the registry. The stakeholder may also be the party that will require the data, including regulatory authorities. Industry or private foundation funders of studies are typically referred to as sponsors, while commonly used terms for government funders include funding agency or contracting agency.

EXPLANATION

The Primary Stakeholder(s) are the key registry sponsors and champions. They will drive the program's objectives, and often remain heavily involved in the registry's leadership throughout its duration.

ISSUES

Sponsors of a registry, such as pharmaceutical manufacturers, may have additional goals beyond scientific objectives (*see term:* Registry Purpose).

BIBLIOGRAPHY

Chapter 2. Planning a registry. In: Gliklich RE, Dreyer NA, eds. *Registries for Evaluating Patient Outcomes: A User's Guide.* 2nd ed. (Prepared by Outcome DEcIDE Center [Outcome Sciences, Inc. d/b/a Outcome] under contract no. HHSA290200500351 T03.) AHRQ Publication No. 10-EHC049. Rockville, MD: Agency for Healthcare Research and Quality; 2010:23-52.

Berger ML, Bingefors K, Hedblom EC, et al. *Health Care Cost, Quality, and Outcomes: ISPOR Book of Terms.* Lawrenceville, NJ: ISPOR; 2003.

Secondary Stakeholders

BRIEF DEFINITION

Those individuals or groups that are not directly involved with the registry. They include regulators, reimbursement committees, Health Technology Assessment (HTA) organizations, treating physicians and their patients, and professional or patient societies that can use the data and/or will be impacted by the findings.

EXPLANATION

Secondary stakeholders are an integral part of any registry, as they may have significant input into the type and scope of data to be collected. Experience shows that their close involvement significantly increases the chances of running a successful registry and producing good quality data, enhancing acceptance by all stakeholders.

VALUE AND USE

Consideration of the final purpose of registry data and the different secondary stakeholders, to whom information based on the registry data are to be presented, can help to more tightly define core data elements and the targeted quality of the data in terms of completeness and accuracy.

ISSUES

Not all the variables of interest to secondary stakeholders may be captured in the registry.

BIBLIOGRAPHY

Chapter 2. Planning a registry. In: Gliklich RE, Dreyer NA, eds. *Registries for Evaluating Patient Outcomes: A User's Guide.* 2nd ed. (Prepared by Outcome DEcIDE Center [Outcome Sciences, Inc. d/b/a Outcome] under contract no. HHSA290200500351 T03.) AHRQ Publication No. 10-EHC049. Rockville, MD: Agency for Healthcare Research and Quality; 2010:23-52.

Governance and Oversight

BRIEF DEFINITION

Guidance and high-level decision making, including concept, funding, execution, and dissemination of information.

EXPLANATION

Registry governance and oversight functions could include any or all of the following: executive, scientific, liaison with all stakeholders, adjudication, drug safety monitoring, data access, data use and publications. The team should include clinicians or experts that monitor registry outcomes, regulations, and safety, as well as representatives of the sponsoring organization; the overall aim is to support program strategic governance and execution. Specific requirements and guidelines in relevant countries and for relevant stakeholders (eg, Food and Drug Administration [FDA], National Health Service [NHS], sponsor organizations) should be reviewed and followed (*see term:* Evaluating and Ensuring Registry Quality).

VALUE AND USE

Ensuring sound registry governance is key to the program's success. The governance structure should allow for ongoing oversight of registry operations, decision making and outcomes, and also ensure transparency in these to stakeholders.

ISSUES

Registry governance must be robust enough to provide appropriate oversight and guidance, without adding undue complexity, or obstacles to the registry's progress.

BIBLIOGRAPHY

Chapter 2. Planning a registry. In: Gliklich RE, Dreyer NA, eds. *Registries for Evaluating Patient Outcomes: A User's Guide*. 2nd ed. (Prepared by Outcome DEcIDE Center [Outcome Sciences, Inc. d/b/a Outcome] under contract no. HHSA290200500351 T03.) AHRQ Publication No. 10-EHC049. Rockville, MD: Agency for Healthcare Research and Quality; 2010:23-52.

GOV.UK. Department of Health. Research Governance Framework for Health and Social Care: second edition. https://www.gov.uk/government/uploads/system/uploads/attachment_data/file/139565/dh_4122427.pdf. Published April 24, 2005. Accessed April 25, 2013.

Scientific Advisory Board (SAB)

BRIEF DEFINITION

Academic, governmental and other independent experts who provide technical advice directly to the sponsor and/or contract research organization (CRO).

EXPLANATION

The SAB may include experts in areas ranging from database content, clinical research, clinical practice, epidemiology, and/or biostatistics. The SAB is engaged throughout the registry to advise on program design and operations, and, often, to identify and facilitate registry analyses and publications.

VALUE AND USE

Through input from the SAB, the sponsor and CRO seek to enhance the quality and credibility of the registry.

ISSUES

To be effective, SABs must be independent and perceived to be free of any significant conflict of interest, and must be uncompromised by bias (*see term:* Conflict of Interest). Members are typically participating in the registry, but participation is not mandatory. SABs should also be properly balanced, allowing for a spectrum of views and appropriate expertise, and should reflect the overall participation in the registry. For example, if the registry sites include both academic and community-based sites, the SAB should include both academic and community-based advisors.

BIBLIOGRAPHY

Chapter 2. Planning a registry. In: Gliklich RE, Dreyer NA, eds. *Registries for Evaluating Patient Outcomes: A User's Guide*. 2nd ed. (Prepared by Outcome DEcIDE Center [Outcome Sciences, Inc. d/b/a Outcome] under contract no. HHSA290200500351 T03.) AHRQ Publication No. 10-EHC049. Rockville, MD: Agency for Healthcare Research and Quality; 2010:23-52.

Data Ownership and Access Rights

BRIEF DEFINITION

Exclusive rights, control, and access to the data elements within a registry.

EXPLANATION

Data ownership refers to both the possession of and responsibility for information. Ownership implies power and control. The control of information includes the right to assign not just access privileges to others but also the ability to modify, package, sell or remove data. The funding of a registry can sometimes lead to contracts for data access.

VALUE AND USE

Data ownership and access are central to the design and conduct of a registry, as it will control how the registry's data are used, and therefore what value the registry will ultimately provide to its stakeholders.

ISSUES

As there are no widely accepted social or legal standards currently governing property rights in health information, claims of ownership for registries may be made by a variety of involved parties. In theory, copyright protection for patient information held in registries may be claimed but this has not been legally tested. Multiple entities are positioned to assert ownership claims to health information in various forms. These include health care providers and insurance plans, funding agencies for registry projects, research institutions, government agencies, and biopharmaceutical/device manufacturers.

Individuals, including patients, registry developers, and investigators may also assert ownership claims to health information. As health information moves from its creation to different uses, the rights of ownership may be transferred (assigned), shared, or maintained, with use of the information licensed. Presently, in each of these transactions, the rights of ownership are negotiated on a case-by-case basis. Data access and publication policies for a registry should be established at an early stage (*see term:* Record Retention and Database Archiving).

BIBLIOGRAPHY

Chapter 2. Planning a registry. In: Gliklich RE, Dreyer NA, eds. *Registries for Evaluating Patient Outcomes: A User's Guide*. 2nd ed. (Prepared by Outcome DEcIDE Center [Outcome Sciences, Inc. d/b/a Outcome] under contract no. HHSA290200500351 T03.) AHRQ Publication No. 10-EHC049. Rockville, MD: Agency for Healthcare Research and Quality; 2010:23-52.

Surveillance, Epidemiology, and End Results. National Cancer Institute. http://seer.cancer.gov/data/. Accessed April 24, 2013.

Ethics and Privacy

Belmont Report (Public Law 93-348 [1974], Title II)

BRIEF DEFINITION

Ethics and privacy issues relating to human subjects in clinical trials have been defined in the *Belmont Report*. This historical document provides the moral framework for understanding regulations in the US on the use of humans in experimental research. It outlines 3 major ethical principles: Respect for Persons, Beneficence, and Justice, and their applications in informed consent, assessment of risks and benefits, and selection of subjects, respectively.

EXPLANATION

The *Belmont Report* was created by the former United States Department of Health, Education, and Welfare, later renamed Health and Human Services (HHS). It is entitled *Ethical Principles and Guidelines for the Protection of Human Subjects of Research*, and serves as the US interpretation or representation of the Nuremburg Code. It was created April 18, 1979, and gets its name from the Belmont Conference Center where it was drafted. This report also formed the foundation of a 1991 issuance of the Common Rule regulations, a uniform set of rules for the protection of human subjects (*see term:* Common Rule).

VALUE AND USE

In patient registries, as in all observational research, the protocol does not dictate treatment and does not introduce any investigational (ie, not-yet-approved by regulatory authorities) treatment to registry participants. Therefore, ethical concerns in patient registries center more on data privacy as a result of registry participation than on any concerns with the treatments that patients are receiving in everyday care.

BIBLIOGRAPHY

The Belmont Report. Office of the Secretary. Ethical Principles and Guidelines for the Protection of Human Subjects of Research. The National Commission for the Protection of Human Subjects of Biomedical and Behavioral Research. US Department of Health and Human Services. http://www.hhs.gov/ohrp/humansubjects/guidance/belmont.html. Published April 18, 1979. Accessed April 24, 2013.

Council for International Organizations of Medical Sciences (CIOMS). International Ethical Guidelines for Biomedical Research Involving Human Subjects. http://www.cioms.ch/publications/layout_guide2002.pdf. Published 2002. Accessed April 24, 2013.

CIOMS International Guidelines for Ethical Review of Epidemiological Studies. http://www.cioms.ch/publications/guidelines/1991_texts_of_guidelines.htm. Published 1991. Accessed April 24, 2013.

Zimmerman JF. The Belmont report: an ethical framework for protecting research subject. *The ACRP Monitor.* 1997. http://www.impactcg.com/docs/BelmontReport.pdf. Accessed April 24, 2013.

» *Respect for Persons*

BRIEF DEFINITION

Respecting the autonomy of every individual and the opportunity for all subjects to obtain and warrant the proper informed consent.

EXPLANATION

The European Union (EU) Clinical Trials Directive, which aims at improving the protection of patients, strictly regulates how a trial should be performed and how consent should be obtained from the participants. Similarly, the *Belmont Report* provides the moral framework for understanding regulations in the USA on the use of humans in experimental research (*see term:* Belmont Report).

VALUE AND USE

Participation in a registry requires the consent of the patient (*see term:* Informed Consent), which also implies informing about the benefits as well as the potential adverse effects of usual care.

ISSUES

As noninterventional studies are not within the scope of the regulations, the same regulations would not apply to patient registries considered purely observational in nature. However, if patient-reported outcome assessments, or other assessments required for registry participants, are considered as an intervention, a patient registry would fall under the requirements of the EU Clinical Trials Directive. Currently there are no generally accepted criteria for determining when additional diagnostic and monitoring procedures should be considered interventional. This issue remains one that has to be decided on a case-by-case basis for individual registries.

BIBLIOGRAPHY

The Belmont Report. Office of the Secretary. Ethical Principles and Guidelines for the Protection of Human Subjects of Research. The National Commission for the Protection of Human Subjects of Biomedical and Behavioral Research. US Department of Health and Human Services. http://www.hhs.gov/ohrp/humansubjects/guidance/belmont.html. Published April 18, 1979. Accessed April 24, 2013.

European Commission. *Directive 2001/20/EC of the European Parliament and of the Council of 4 April 2001 on the Approximation of the Laws, Regulations and Administrative Provisions of the Member States Relating to the Implementation of Good Clinical Practice in the Conduct of Clinical Trials on Medicinal Products for Human Use.* http://www.eortc.be/services/doc/clinical-eu-directive-04-april-01.pdf. Accessed April 24, 2013.

» *Beneficence*

BRIEF DEFINITION

Beneficence refers to maximizing benefits of the study while in turn minimizing risks to the patient.

EXPLANATION

Beneficence is mainly an issue in interventional trials. In an observational study, the benefits and potential risks to the patient are not related to a treatment or intervention determined by a study protocol, but reflect health care as commonly practiced.

VALUE AND USE

Participation in a registry requires the consent of the patient, which also implies providing information to the patient about the benefits and potential adverse effects of usual care (*see term:* Informed Consent).

ISSUES

Because patients are treated with routine practice in patient registries, the treatment benefits derived by the patient are no greater than what they would be if the patient was not participating in the registry. However, the patient may derive benefits or satisfaction from participating in the study if the patient feels that he or she is contributing to research and the common good. This same benefit may be derived by the registry sites, although the site may derive additional study benefit from receiving information on how their site is performing (both in terms of study outputs such as patients enrolled and completed, as well as in terms of patient outcomes) against collective benchmarks for the other sites in the registry.

BIBLIOGRAPHY

The Belmont Report. Office of the Secretary. Ethical Principles and Guidelines for the Protection of Human Subjects of Research. The National Commission for the Protection of Human Subjects of Biomedical and Behavioral Research. US Department of Health and Human Services. http://www.hhs.gov/ohrp/humansubjects/guidance/belmont.html. Published April 18, 1979. Accessed April 24, 2013.

» *Justice*

BRIEF DEFINITION

The concept of justice in medical research requires that risks and benefits of research should be fairly distributed, and that groups and individuals participating in research should share the potential to benefit from study findings. Certain governing or regulatory bodies have ethical/legal provisions to ensure that certain subgroups of people are adequately represented in clinical research, such as women and minority populations.

EXPLANATION

Historically, much medical and biological research has been conducted on groups selected for convenience or inability to protest (eg, prisoners, racial and ethnic minorities, institutionalized persons, and the poor and disenfranchised). The *Belmont Report*, and other ethical principles, was developed to respond to this situation, and bar such exploitative practices (*see term:* Belmont Report).

VALUE AND USE

Because registries are observational in design, justice is less of an issue in registries than it is in interventional trials. Registry participants typically receive usual care and, unlike interventional trials, are not randomly assigned to comparator treatments which may include placebo or other less studied treatments. As a result, the risk and/or benefit of participating in a registry is far less than that of an interventional trial. Since patient registries attempt to be representative of the population, the risk of disproportionate benefit or risk is not a consideration.

BIBLIOGRAPHY

The Belmont Report. Office of the Secretary. Ethical Principles and Guidelines for the Protection of Human Subjects of Research. The National Commission for the Protection of Human Subjects of Biomedical and Behavioral Research. US Department of Health and Human Services. http://www.hhs.gov/ohrp/humansubjects/guidance/belmont.html. Published April 18, 1979. Accessed April 24, 2013.

Friedman LM, Furberg CD, DeMets DL. *Fundamentals of Clinical Trials*. New York, NY: Springer; 1998.

Informed Consent

BRIEF DEFINITION

A legal document representing the agreement for a patient's proposed participation in a study, and any accompanying medical treatment or nontreatment, in a language that the patient can clearly understand.

EXPLANATION
Obtaining informed patient consent in experimental studies requires researchers to disclose the benefits, risks, and alternatives to the proposed study treatment or nontreatment.

VALUE AND USE
The purpose of the informed consent in a registry is not to inform about any risk in participating, as it does not include an experimental treatment. But the patient needs to be informed about the purpose of collecting the data, how the data will be handled and who is going to see the data.

ISSUES
When creating a registry, consent is required for access to and the use of any identifiable or potentially identifiable data which is going to be collected; however, there is no consistent guidance at an international level for obtaining this consent. Requiring explicit written consent may be an unrealistic requirement for a study which relies heavily on retrospective data, and, at least in the US, consent is typically not required where the data will be anonymized. Upon institutional review board (IRB) or ethics committee review, exemption from review or waiver of informed consent may be granted in such cases. A waiver of informed or written consent is more common in studies where the protocol describes analysis of preexisting data (ie, retrospective studies). However, in some cases informed consent may still be required for retrospective chart review, depending on what consent was defined when the database was established (*see term:* Institutional Review Board/Ethical Committee Approval).

In Europe, requirements for informed consent may differ. For instance, as long as the physician retains a key code for reidentifying the data, the data is not defined as anonymous according to the EU Data Protection act.

BIBLIOGRAPHY
Ingelfinger JR, Drazen JM. Registry research and medical privacy. *N Engl J Med*. 2004;350: 1452-1453.

Correspondence. Registries and informed consent. *N Engl J Med*. 2004;351:612-614.

Common Rule

BRIEF DEFINITION
A US federal policy regarding human subject protection that applies to 17 federal agencies and offices. However, it does not apply to federal agencies that have not signed the agreement (eg, Department of Labor, etc.).

EXPLANATION

The main elements of the Common Rule include requirements for assuring compliance by research institutions, requirements for researchers' obtaining and documenting informed consent, and requirements for IRB membership, function, operations, review of research, and record keeping.

BIBLIOGRAPHY

U.S. Department of Health and Human Services. Title 45 Public Welfare. Subpart A. Part 46 Protection of Human Subjects. http://www.hhs.gov/ohrp/humansubjects/guidance/45cfr46.html. Updated January 15, 2009. Accessed April 24, 2013.

Chapter 8. Principles of registry ethics, data ownership, and privacy. In: Gliklich RE, Dreyer NA, eds. *Registries for Evaluating Patient Outcomes: A User's Guide*. 2nd ed. (Prepared by Outcome DEcIDE Center [Outcome Sciences, Inc. d/b/a Outcome] under contract no. HHSA290200500351 T03.) AHRQ Publication No. 10-EHC049. Rockville, MD: Agency for Healthcare Research and Quality; 2010:167-204.

Institutional Review Board (IRB)/Ethical Committee Approval

BRIEF DEFINITION

A group that has been formally designated to approve, monitor, and review research that involves humans with the aim of protecting the rights and welfare of those subjects.

EXPLANATION

An IRB/institutional ethics committee (IEC) performs critical oversight functions for research conducted on human subjects to ensure, as far as possible, that the research is scientifically sound, ethical, and in accordance with regulatory requirements. IRB or IEC approval represents the confirmation from a medical review board that the study poses no undue risk to the patient, that the informed consent is understandable and that the study does not prevent the physician from meeting his or her obligations to the patient. As registries are observational studies, it is sometimes possible for IRB/IEC boards to grant an expedited review of the registry protocol, which can save time on the start-up of the registry.

VALUE AND USE

As with all research involving human subjects, IRB or IEC review is required for registry-based research, and the fact that approval was obtained and the manner in which informed consent was obtained (ie, oral or written) should be noted in the Methods section of all publications stemming from registry data. In most cases, biomedical journals now require such a statement for all studies conducted with human participants (International Committee of Medical Journal Authors [ICMJE] uniform requirements [*see term:* Reporting and Dissemination of Registry-Based Studies]).

ISSUES

If patient-reported outcome assessments, or other assessments required for registry participants, are considered by the IRB or IEC as nonstandard or outside the realm of usual care, the IRB or IEC may deem these assessments to be an intervention, particularly if the results are fed back to the physician treating the patient and thus potentially altering the course of usual care in the absence of those assessments. In this case, a patient registry would be considered an interventional study and fall under the requirements of the EU Clinical Trials Directive. Currently there are no generally accepted criteria for determining when additional diagnostic and monitoring procedures should be considered interventional. This issue remains one that has to be decided on a case-by-case basis for individual registries. Complicating matters is that in multicountry patient registries, such assessments may be considered interventional in one country but not in another.

The reporting of ethical approval and patient consent in published studies has improved in recent years, but is still lacking for study designs, other than RCTs, including cohorts, cross-sectional studies, and analyses of routine data. Where space constraints in print journals do not permit complete discussion of patient consent or ethics review procedures, internet appendices should be used to make this information available.

BIBLIOGRAPHY

McFadden E. *Management of Data in Clinical Trials*. New York, NY: John Wiley & Sons, Inc; 1998.

National Institute on Drug Abuse. *Guidelines for Developing a Data and Safety Monitoring Plan*. http://www.nida.nih.gov/Funding/DSMBSOP.html. Accessed April 24, 2013.

National Institutes of Health. *NIH guide: NIH Policy for Data and Safety Monitoring*. http://grants.nih.gov/grants/guide/notice-files/not98-084.html. Published June 10, 1998. Accessed April 24, 2013.

Redshaw ME, Harris A, Baum JD. Research ethics committee audit: differences between committees. *J Med Ethics*. 1996;22:78-82.

Swerdlow PS. Use of humans in biomedical experimentation. In: Macrina FL, ed. *Scientific Integrity: An Introductory Text with Cases*. Washington, DC: ASM Press; 1995.

International Committee of Medical Journal Editors. Uniform Requirements for Manuscripts Submitted to Biomedical Journals: Writing and Editing for Biomedical Publications. http://www.icmje.org/. Updated April 2010. Accessed April 18, 2013.

Schroter S, Plowman R, Hutchings A, Gonzalez A. Reporting ethics committee approval and patient consent by study design in five general medical journals. *J Med Ethics*. 2006;32:718-732.

World Health Organization. Operational Guidelines for Ethics Committees That Review Biomedical Research. http://www.who.int/tdr/publications/training-guideline-publications/operational-guidelines-ethics-biomedical-research/en/. Geneva, Switzerland: WHO. Published 2000. Accessed April 24, 2013.

Council for International Organization of Medical Sciences (CIOMS) International Guidelines for Ethical Review of Epidemiological Studies

BRIEF DEFINITION

CIOMS is an international nongovernmental organization that works closely with the World Health Organization (WHO). It was founded under the auspices of WHO and the United Nations Educational, Scientific and Cultural Organization (UNESCO) in 1949.

EXPLANATION

The guidelines identify how individuals should respond to any ethical issues that are raised by the process of producing information on the distribution and determinants of health-related states or events in specified populations.

VALUE AND USE

Ethical guidance for epidemiologists, sponsors, reviewers and study participants in epidemiological studies.

BIBLIOGRAPHY

CIOMS International Ethical Guidelines for Biomedical Research Involving Human Subjects. http://www.cioms.ch/publications/layout_guide2002.pdf. Published 2002. Accessed April 24, 2013.

CIOMS International Guidelines for Ethical Review of Epidemiological Studies. http://www.cioms.ch/publications/guidelines/1991_texts_of_guidelines.htm. Published 1991. Accessed April 24, 2013.

Declaration of Helsinki

BRIEF DEFINITION

The *Declaration of Helsinki* was adopted by the World Medical Association in 1964 and has since been revised 6 times. This declaration was the first internationally recognized statement of ethical principles for medical research involving human subjects, including research on identifiable human material and data.

EXPLANATION

The *Helsinki Declaration* forms the basis for several other documents, including the International Conference on Harmonization (ICH), the EMEA ICH *Clinical Trial Directive* and the Oviedo Convention (*see term:* International Conference on Harmonization [ICH]; Good Clinical Practice [GCP]).

VALUE AND USE
The *Helsinki Declaration* primarily concerns experimental trials, but the rules regarding informed consent are also applicable to a patient registry and noninterventional studies.

BIBLIOGRAPHY
Kimmelman J, Weijer C, Meslin EM. Helsinki discords: FDA, ethics, and international drug trials. *Lancet*. 2009;373:13-14.

The Declaration of Helsinki: Ethical Principles for Medical Research Involving Human Subjects. World Medical Association. http://www.wma.net/en/30publications/10policies/b3/index.html. Accessed April 24, 2013.

International Conference on Harmonization (ICH): Good Clinical Practice (GCP)

BRIEF DEFINITION
The international ethical and scientific quality standard for the conduct of clinical trials involving human subjects agreed to by the ICH in May 1996. *Good Clinical Practice (GCP)* guidelines give standards on the conduct of clinical trials. They also define the roles and responsibilities of clinical trial sponsors and clinical research investigators.

EXPLANATION
The purpose of the ICH is to make recommendations on ways to harmonize the interpretation and application of technical guidelines and requirements for product registration in order to minimize the need to duplicate the testing carried out during the research and development of new medicines. This is achieved by maintaining a forum for a constructive dialogue between regulatory authorities and the pharmaceutical industry on the real and perceived differences in the technical requirements for product registration in the EU, USA and Japan in order to ensure a timelier introduction of new medicinal products, and their availability to patients. GCP is an international quality standard provided by ICH. The GCP guidelines include standards on how clinical trials should be conducted and define the roles and responsibilities of clinical trial sponsors, clinical research investigators, and monitors.

VALUE AND USE
Although the GCP guidelines are mainly focused on clinical trials, the ethical principles regarding the rights of the study participant, informed consent and storing of study data also apply to patient registries. Aspects of ICH-GCP in many, but not all countries, serve as guidance for observational studies in clinical settings.

ISSUES

Not all aspects of GCPs are applicable to patient registries.

BIBLIOGRAPHY

International Conference on Harmonisation. http://www.ich.org. Accessed April 24, 2013.

U.S. Food and Drug Administration. Rules, Guidance and Recommendations. http://www.fda.gov/cber/guidelines.htm. Accessed April 24, 2013.

Benson K, Hartz AJ. A comparison of observational studies and randomized, controlled trials. *N Engl J Med.* 2000;342:1878-1886.

Concato J, Shah N, Horwitz RI. Randomized, controlled trials, observational studies, and the hierarchy of research designs. *N Engl J Med.* 2000;342:1887-1892.

U.S. National Institutes of Health. Understanding clinical trials. http://clinicaltrials.gov/ct2/info/understand. Updated August 2012. Accessed April 24, 2013.

US Food and Drug Administration (FDA) Regulations

BRIEF DEFINITION

Regulations for conduct of a clinical trial or registry.

EXPLANATION

Several regulations governing clinical trials may also be relevant to registries, even though these observational studies are not evaluating investigational drugs or devices. These regulations can be located in Chapter 21 of the *Code of Federal Regulations (CFR).*

VALUE AND USE

Ensure industry compliance with patient safety related to handling of relationships between study sponsors and investigators, informed consent and privacy rights of patients, and reporting of AEs in postmarketing safety commitment studies that are observational.

BIBLIOGRAPHY

U.S. Food and Drug Administration. Federal Food, Drug, and Cosmetic Act of 1938 (21 USC §301-95). http://www.fda.gov/default.htm. Accessed April 24, 2013.

U.S. Food and Drug Administration. Code of Federal Regulations (CFR). 21CFR part 11. http://www.accessdata.fda.gov/scripts/cdrh/cfdocs/cfcfr/cfrsearch.cfm?cfrpart=11. Accessed April 24, 2013.

Office of Inspector General, U.S. Department of Health and Human Services. Federal Anti-Kickback Law and Regulatory Safe Harbors: Fact Sheet. http://oig.hhs.gov/fraud/docs/safeharbor-regulations/safefs.htm. Published November 1999. Accessed April 24, 2013.

U.S. Food and Drug Administration. FDA Adverse Event Reporting System (FAERS). http://www.fda.gov/Drugs/GuidanceComplianceRegulatoryInformation/Surveillance/AdverseDrugEffects/default.htm. Updated September 10, 2013. Accessed April 24, 2013.

Conflict of Interest

BRIEF DEFINITION

Any relationship with an individual, organization, or company that may have the potential to introduce bias, alter final study results, or impact reporting and disclosure of results. This may include financial and/or material support for one or more aspects of the study (registry initiation, data collection, analyses, or manuscript/abstract/presentation writing).

EXPLANATION

In order to reduce conflicts of interest, the FDA requires a clinical investigator to certify that no financial arrangements with a registry sponsor have been made where study outcome could affect compensation; that the investigator has no proprietary interest in the tested product; that the investigator does not have a significant equity interest in the sponsor of the covered study, and; that the investigator has not received significant payments of other sorts.

VALUE AND USE

Increasingly, individual studies receive funding from commercial firms, private foundations, and government. The conditions of this funding have the potential to bias and otherwise discredit the research.

Financial relationships among industry, scientific investigators, and academic institutions are widespread. Conflicts of interest arising from these ties can influence biomedical research in important ways. Disclosure of the sponsorship informs consumers of the research regarding potential bias and influence. Disclosure of sponsorship is required for publication or presentation of study results; in addition, sponsors should impose no impediment, direct or indirect, on publication of the study's full results. Asserting the absence of conflict of interest gives credibility to the registry's results.

ISSUES

Conflict of interest and the influence of industry sponsorship on science are topics of much discussion in the biomedical field as a whole. Ethical conduct standards for researchers have been developed and promulgated by many scientific societies, including ISPOR.

Financial conflicts of interest on the part of investigators conducting a study may compromise the well-being of research subjects and impede the publication of important data, causing publication bias (*see term:* Publication Bias). As any investigator participating in a product registry is aware of the existence of the registry, and the compensation to his or her practice for enrolling a patient in that registry, before and at the time of prescribing a treatment to a patient (ie, overt nature of prospective research), a physician participating in a registry may, on the margin, be more likely to prescribe the product under study in the registry than a product not under study in that product registry. To the extent that this occurs, this conflict of interest may somewhat compromise the real-world nature of physician prescribing patterns observed in the registry.

BIBLIOGRAPHY

U.S. Department of Health and Human Services. Guidance for Clinical Investigators, Industry, and FDA Staff Financial Disclosure by Clinical Investigators. http://www.fda.gov/downloads/RegulatoryInformation/Guidances/UCM341008.pdf. Published February 2013. Accessed April 24, 2013.

Bekelman JE, Li Y, Gross CP. Scope and impact of financial conflicts of interest in biomedical research: a systematic review. *JAMA*. 2003;289:454-465.

Studdert DM, Mello MM, Brennan TA. Financial conflicts of interest in physicians' relationships with the pharmaceutical industry – self regulation in the shadow of federal prosecution. *N Eng J Med*. 2004;351:1891-1900.

Rochon PA, Hoey J, Chan AW, et al. Financial conflicts of interest checklist 2010 for clinical research studies. *Open Med*. 2010;4:e69-e91.

International Committee of Medical Journal Editors. Uniform Requirements for Manuscripts Submitted to Biomedical Journals: Writing and Editing for Biomedical Publications. http://www.icmje.org/. Updated April 2010. Accessed April 18, 2013.

Lexchin J, Bero LA, Djulbegovic B, Clark O. Pharmaceutical industry sponsorship and research outcome and quality: systematic review. *BMJ*. 2003;326:1167-1170.

ISPOR Code of Ethics. International Society for Pharmacoeconomics and Outcomes Research. http://www.ispor.org/workpaper/CodeOfEthics.asp. Published March 2008. Accessed April 24, 2013.

Data Privacy and Committees

BRIEF DEFINITION

Data privacy encompasses the relationship between collection and dissemination of data on study participants, the public expectation of privacy, and the legal and political issues surrounding these concepts. Often a committee is established to advise on programmatic, policy, operational, administrative, and/or technological issues within the study that relate to personally identifiable information, as well as data integrity and other privacy-related matters (such as data access [*see term:* Data Ownership and Access Rights]).

EXPLANATION

Privacy concerns exist wherever personally identifiable information is collected and stored—in digital form or otherwise. Given these concerns, standards for safeguarding the privacy of this information against inappropriate release have been established (for example the Health Insurance Portability and Accountability Act [HIPAA] Privacy Rule in the United States [*see term:* HIPAA]).

VALUE AND USE

Privacy committees can ensure that privacy is a fundamental consideration while collecting and using personally identifiable information in research. The deidentification of data can help ensure data privacy and answer the concerns of ethics and review boards overseeing clinical research. With regard to publication of results from registry-based research, as with all research based on human participants, individually identifiable health information must not be disclosed unless a signed statement of informed consent to publish has been obtained. Informed consent to publish should be obtained from all persons (parents or legal guardians for minors) who can be recognized (including by the patients themselves) in written descriptions, photographs, or pedigrees. Such persons should be shown the manuscript before its submission as a part of gaining their consent. In some cases journals require this consent to be submitted along with the manuscript.

ISSUES

Improper or nonexistent disclosure can be the root cause of privacy issues. Maintaining confidentially/data privacy throughout the research process has become increasingly critical given the electronic availability of individually identifiable health information.

BIBLIOGRAPHY

Europa. Summaries of EU legislation. European Parliament and Council Directive 95/46/EC of 24 October 1995 on the protection of individuals with regard to the processing of personal data and on the free movement of such data (Official Journal L 281 of 23.11.1995). http://europa.eu/legislation_summaries/information_society/data_protection/l14012_en.htm. Updated February 1, 2011. Accessed April 24, 2013.

Department of Health and Human Services. Office of the Secretary. 45 CFR Parts 160 and 164. HIPAA Administrative Simplification: Enforcement; Final Rule. Federal Register Vol 71;32. http://www.gpo.gov/fdsys/pkg/FR-2006-02-16/html/06-1376.htm. Published February 16, 2006. Accessed April 24, 2013.

International Committee of Medical Journal Editors. Uniform Requirements for Manuscripts Submitted to Biomedical Journals. http://www.icmje.org/. Updated April 2010. Accessed May 1, 2013.

Deidentified Information

BRIEF DEFINITION

Health care information from which any detail that identifies, or provides a reasonable basis to believe it can be used to identify, an individual has been removed.

EXPLANATION

Patient identifiers include any subset of health information, including demographic information that could be used to identify the individual. This personal health information (PHI) includes age, date of birth, home address, physician names.

VALUE AND USE

Deidentification of data helps to ensure data privacy. In patient registries, risk to the patient has more to do with data privacy than with the treatment being observed. Hence, many patients invited to participate in a registry may grant informed consent only if they can be assured that their data will be deidentified to those analyzing the compiled data. However, deidentified data has its largest application in registries linked to medical records. In medical records, deidentified means that the personal identifiers in a record have been extracted and that it would be very difficult to re-establish the identity of any of the persons mentioned in the original record. Unlike anonymized data, where all of the links between a person and the person's record have been irreversibly broken so that it would be virtually impossible to re-establish any of the people in the original record, deidentified patient record data may be reidentified using one of a number of different methods, so long as the IRB/IEC has granted approval. This allows for linkages to patient registry data and therefore an expansion of the observed patient with respect to data elements, settings of care, and time.

ISSUES

Deidentified information may hinder linkage with existing data sources (for instance, as a contingency to missing data for individuals lost to follow-up).

BIBLIOGRAPHY

Europa. Summaries of EU legislation. European Parliament and Council Directive 95/46/EC of 24 October 1995 on the protection of individuals with regard to the processing of personal data and on the free movement of such data (Official Journal L 281 of 23.11.1995). http://europa.eu/legislation_summaries/information_society/data_protection/l14012_en.htm. Updated February 1, 2011. Accessed April 24, 2013.

Department of Health and Human Services. Office of the Secretary. 45 CFR Parts 160 and 164. HIPAA Administrative Simplification: Enforcement; Final Rule. Federal Register Vol 71;32. http://www.gpo.gov/fdsys/pkg/FR-2006-02-16/html/06-1376.htm. Published February 16, 2006. Accessed April 24, 2013.

Chapter 8. Principles of registry ethics, data ownership, and privacy. In: Gliklich RE, Dreyer NA, eds. *Registries for Evaluating Patient Outcomes: A User's Guide*. 2nd ed. (Prepared by Outcome DEcIDE Center [Outcome Sciences, Inc. d/b/a Outcome] under contract no. HHSA290200500351 T03.) AHRQ Publication No. 10-EHC049. Rockville, MD: Agency for Healthcare Research and Quality; 2010:167-204.

United States Government Accountability Office. Report to Congressional Requesters. Health Information Technology. Early Efforts Initiated but Comprehensive Privacy Approach Needed for National Strategy. GAO-07-238. http://www.gao.gov/new.items/d07238.pdf. Published January 2007. Accessed April 24, 2013.

United States Government Accountability Office. Report to Congressional Requesters. Privacy: Alternatives Exist for Enhancing Protection of Personally Identifiable Information. GAO-08-536. http://www.gao.gov/new.items/d08536.pdf. Published May 2008. Accessed April 24, 2013.

Data Protection

BRIEF DEFINITION

Measures taken to safeguard the anonymity of patients and limit access to viewing the data; examples include deidentification of patient identifying information and data transfer using secured files that are password protected.

EXPLANATION

To respect the privacy of patients, internal procedures need to be enacted to review and monitor the use of patient data to ensure that it is used responsibly and complies with internationally recognized standards of privacy protection. Internationally recognized standards include, but are not limited to, the European Union Data Protection Directive [EC/95/46], the US HIPAA, and the US Department of Commerce Safe Harbor Agreement. Such standards require that the processing of personal data, both automated and manual, meet the following basic principles of data protection:

- Data is fairly and lawfully processed;
- Data is processed for limited and explicit purposes;
- Data use is adequate, relevant, and not excessive;
- Data is kept current (when necessary) and accurate;
- Data is not kept longer than necessary;
- Data processing is in accordance with the rights of data subjects;
- Data is secured;
- Data is not transferred to third parties unless an adequate level of data protection precautions exist.

VALUE AND USE

Data protection is a secure measure against potential abuses of the privacy of patient's health information (*see term:* Data Ownership and Access Rights).

ISSUES

Data protection and privacy requirements differ from country to country.

BIBLIOGRAPHY

Data protection officer. European Commission. http://ec.europa.eu/dataprotectionofficer/index_en.htm. Accessed April 24, 2013.

The Health Insurance Portability and Accountability Act of 1996 (HIPAA) privacy and security rules. U.S. Department of Health and Human Services. http://www.hhs.gov/ocr/privacy. Accessed September 7, 2011.

Europa. Summaries of EU legislation. European Parliament and Council Directive 95/46/EC of 24 October 1995 on the protection of individuals with regard to the processing of personal data and on the free movement of such data (Official Journal L 281 of 23.11.1995). http://europa.eu/legislation_summaries/information_society/data_protection/l14012_en.htm. Updated February 1, 2011. Accessed April 24, 2013.

U.S.-EU Safe Harbor Overview. Expert.gov. http://export.gov/safeharbor/eu/eg_main_018476.asp. Updated April 26, 2012. Accessed April 24, 2013.

United States Government Accountability Office. Report to Congressional Requesters. Health Information Technology. Early Efforts Initiated but Comprehensive Privacy Approach Needed for National Strategy. GAO-07-238. http://www.gao.gov/new.items/d07238.pdf. Published January 2007. Accessed April 24, 2013.

United States Government Accountability Office. Report to Congressional Requesters. Privacy: Alternatives Exist for Enhancing Protection of Personally Identifiable Information. GAO-08-536. http://www.gao.gov/new.items/d08536.pdf. Published May 2008. Accessed April 24, 2013.

Privacy Rule/US Health Insurance Portability and Accountability Act (HIPAA)

BRIEF DEFINITION

A provision within HIPAA called the Privacy Rule represents the first comprehensive federal protection for the privacy of personal health information.

EXPLANATION

HIPAA and its implementing regulations ensure legal protection for the privacy of individually identifiable health information created and maintained by health care providers, health plans, and health care clearing houses. HIPAA permits the use or disclosure of patient information for a registry, subject to specific conditions and in the following circumstances: (1) registries serving public health activities, including registries developed in connection with FDA-regulated products; (2) registries developed for the health care operations of health care providers and insurance plans (covered entities under HIPAA); (3) registries using deidentified health information; (4) registries using a limited dataset of patient information that lacks specified direct identifiers; (5) registries using information obtained with patient authorizations, or; (6) registries using information obtained with a waiver of authorization.

VALUE AND USE

In patient registries, risk to the patient has more to do with data privacy than with treatment. Data protection is a secure measure against potential abuses of the privacy of patient's health information.

BIBLIOGRAPHY

Public Law 104-191. Health Insurance Portability and Accountability Act of 1996. http://aspe.hhs.gov/admnsimp/pl104191.htm. Published August 21,1996. Accessed April 24, 2013.

Department of Health and Human Services. Office of the Secretary. 45 CFR Parts 160 and 164. HIPAA Administrative Simplification: Enforcement; Final Rule. Federal Register Vol 71;32. http://www.gpo.gov/fdsys/pkg/FR-2006-02-16/html/06-1376.htm. Published February 16, 2006. Accessed April 24, 2013.

International Guidelines for Ethical Review of Epidemiological Studies. J Law Med Ethics. 1991:19;247-258.

CIOMS International Guidelines for Ethical Review of Epidemiological Studies. http://www.cioms.ch/publications/guidelines/1991_texts_of_guidelines.htm. Published 1991. Accessed April 24, 2013.

Implementation and Operational Considerations

Size

BRIEF DEFINITION

Size can refer to either the number of sites and patients included in a patient registry, or to the volume and complexity of data being collected.

EXPLANATION

The number of sites and patients expected to participate—along with the volume and complexity of data being collected—will affect the scope and budget of the registry as well as the analytical power.

VALUE AND USE

Registries are often larger, including more sites and patients, than typical clinical trials. This additional size often allows registries to evaluate multiple objectives, as well as assist in identifying events and outcomes of lower incidence.

ISSUES

If the patient registry is developed with a well-defined hypothesis, the required size of the registry may be decided by power analysis to determine the sample size required to confirm whether or not a statistical relationship exists between an intervention and an outcome (*see terms:* Analysis Plan; Statistical Significance Under Large Sample Sizes). If no predefined hypothesis is being tested, as is common in registries, then the size of the registry may depend on other circumstances such as the cost of collecting data on a certain number of eligible patients. If the purpose and conditions for the registry are changed during the course of creating the resource, the final sample size may deviate from that originally intended. Similarly, the number of data points being collected will also impact the meaningfulness and relevance of the analysis, but may also affect the feasibility of conducting the registry, as well as the registry's budget. A registry with many and/or complex data fields may contribute to a richer analysis, but may lead to the study being too burdensome or difficult to implement. Conversely, a registry with fewer data fields may be easier to administer, but may not have the depth needed to conduct meaningful analyses.

BIBLIOGRAPHY

Chapter 2. Planning a registry. In: Gliklich RE, Dreyer NA, eds. *Registries for Evaluating Patient Outcomes: A User's Guide*. 2nd ed. (Prepared by Outcome DEcIDE Center [Outcome Sciences, Inc. d/b/a Outcome] under contract no. HHSA290200500351 T03.) AHRQ Publication No. 10-EHC049. Rockville, MD: Agency for Healthcare Research and Quality; 2010:23-52.

Woodward M. Sample size determination. In: Woodward M, ed. *Epidemiology: Study Design and Data Analysis*. 2nd ed. Boca Raton, FL: Chapman & Hall/CRC Press; 2005:329-362.

Budget

BRIEF DEFINITION

An organizational plan stated in monetary terms with a list of all planned expenses and revenues.

EXPLANATION

The budget typically includes all costs associated with collecting data, managing the study, working with sites, analyzing/reporting the data, and compensating the sites and patients as appropriate. These costs generally represent all staff costs, direct and indirect costs related to the registry, supplies, reimbursement (patient and site), IRB fees, website programming/hosting, and CRO fees, as appropriate to the study.

VALUE AND USE

The budget is a critical tool in the design and management of a registry. Describing the costs associated with each element of the registry, and their interdependencies, will provide key support for program-design decisions, and for ongoing management of the registry. Unit costs may, in fact, dictate decisions on the size and duration of the registry, both initially and as the program is evaluated and revised annually throughout its duration.

ISSUES

Registry budgets must be monitored closely and managed throughout the study, to ensure that the program is proceeding as planned and is moving in line with budget projections. Since registry operations and parameters are regularly reviewed and revised, the registry budget must be kept in line with these revisions, and should be viewed as a dynamic, living document.

Feasibility

BRIEF DEFINITION

Likelihood that the organizational, economic and implementation approaches proposed will result in the establishment of a registry fit for the research purpose intended.

EXPLANATION

Process of determining if the registry can be executed based on the specifications required to meet the objectives. Factors associated include determining the population from which recruitment can occur, logistics on operations, budgetary considerations, design, timing and regulation compliance.

VALUE AND USE

The feasibility process is critical to determine the success of the registry in meeting specified objectives. This process should carefully incorporate all facets of the registry to determine likelihood of success.

ISSUES

Organizational considerations include a preliminary assessment of availability and access to appropriate patients and to a core dataset. Economic considerations should include an assessment to determine if adequate funding is available for technology infrastructure and appropriate payments to contributing physicians and/or researchers, while implementation considerations include the completeness and accuracy of the data likely to be available.

BIBLIOGRAPHY

Chapter 2. Planning a registry. In: Gliklich RE, Dreyer NA, eds. *Registries for Evaluating Patient Outcomes: A User's Guide*. 2nd ed. (Prepared by Outcome DEcIDE Center [Outcome Sciences, Inc. d/b/a Outcome] under contract no. HHSA290200500351 T03.) AHRQ Publication No. 10-EHC049. Rockville, MD: Agency for Healthcare Research and Quality; 2010:23-52.

Standard Operating Procedures (SOPs)

BRIEF DEFINITION

Written policies and instructions maintained by sponsors and academic research organizations (AROs)/CROs setting out the standards and processes that will be applicable to the operational conduct of the registry/study.

EXPLANATION

SOPs for a registry describe the processes during planning, conduct, evaluation, and quality management of a noninterventional observational study, including the regular training of all involved participants.

All participants in clinical research, such as, sponsors, clinical investigators, IECs/IRBs, monitors, CROs, should develop and follow written SOPs that define responsibilities, records, and methods to be used for study-related activities. For example, sponsors should prepare SOPs for activities such as, investigator's brochure; developing and updating the protocol; case report forms (CRFs) and other study-related documents/procedures including, but not limited to, standard procedures for reviewing AE reports by medical experts, data analysis by statisticians, shipping, handling, and accounting for all supplies of the investigational product, auditing to determine whether or not monitoring is being appropriately carried out, and ensuring that systems for quality control are operational and effective.

Similarly, clinical investigators should develop SOPs for communicating with the IRB/IEC, obtaining and updating informed consent, reporting AEs, preparing and maintaining adequate records, administering the investigational product, and accounting for and disposing of the investigational product. IRBs/IECs usually develop and follow written SOPs for membership requirements, initial and continuing review, communicating with the investigator(s) and institution, and minimizing or eliminating conflicts of interest. Regulators develop SOPs for reviewing applications and safety reports, conducting GCP inspections (where applicable) and communicating findings to the inspected parties, and establishing an infrastructure for due process and imposing sanctions on parties who violate national/local law or regulations.

Similarly, parties involved in observational research using registries should develop written SOPs for the conduct of registries. There appears to be a significant difference in the design and conduct of observational studies across the biopharmaceutical industry, as some companies rely upon their local marketing affiliates to identify and implement such studies while others use a more centralized approach.

VALUE AND USE

SOPs are essential for quality management of research design and conduct.

ISSUES

A majority of organizations do not have SOPs dedicated to noninterventional observational research design and conduct. Registry-specific SOPs should be developed to guide these studies, rather than utilizing SOPs designed for RCTs.

BIBLIOGRAPHY

World Health Organization. Handbook for Good Clinical Research Practice: Guidance for Implementation. http://ori.hhs.gov/documents/WHOHandbookonGCP04-06.pdf. Published 2002. Accessed April 24, 2013.

Pretesting/Pilot testing

BRIEF DEFINITION

Testing data collection instruments for a registry by implementing the completed form on a small scale, prior to it being finalized for the entire study.

EXPLANATION

Pretesting, or pilot testing, may range from administering a subset of the procedures, CRFs, or assessment tools to a few patients, to a launch of the full study with all data capture systems in a limited number of sites.

VALUE AND USE

The trial run of the CRFs or patient questionnaires on a few sites/patients is intended to ensure that they are readable and understandable and also to assess the time required for completion. Careful pilot testing may also help identify potential problems with data capture for analysis purposes (*see term:* Data Quality Assurance). A library of past CRFs or CRF components maintained by an institution may also be a helpful resource for effective CRF creation.

ISSUES

In addition to testing content and readability, pilot testing may be used to establish appropriate reimbursement rates (ie, fair market value based on usual rates for an average time for completion) for investigators and site staff and also evaluate the overall burden on the site and/or patients. Reimbursement to investigators or patients which is not commensurate with the expected time burden may be seen as an inappropriate incentive by regulatory bodies or ethics committees.

BIBLIOGRAPHY

Theobald K, Capan M, Herbold M, et al. Quality assurance in non-interventional studies. *Ger Med Sci*. 2009;7:Doc29.

Nahm M, Shepherd J, Buzenberg A, et al. Design and implementation of an institutional case report form library. *Clin Trials*. 2011;8:94-102.

Study Population

BRIEF DEFINITION

The universe of patients which is represented by the registry and which the sample enrolled in the registry represent.

EXPLANATION

The study population is the larger group of patients from which the sample of patients eligible and included in the registry, according to the definitions included in the registry protocol, are selected. Inclusion criteria are a set of conditions that prospective subjects must meet to be eligible for participation in a study. Exclusion criteria are conditions which preclude entrance of candidates into the study, even if the inclusion criteria are fulfilled.

VALUE AND USE

The population is the target group of individuals which the registry seeks to better understand. The definition of the population is a key factor in determining the registry sample as these individuals will then represent the broader and larger group of individuals.

ISSUES

The overall study population may need to be differentiated from the analysis population, which, depending on the analysis, can represent different subsets of the study population. For example, while the study population may include all patients enrolled in a patient registry, a safety population may include only those patients who actually received at least one dose of the drug or product under observation. Selection bias can occur in either the selection of patients into the registry from the target population, and/or in selection of analyzable subsets from the overall study population (*see term:* Selection Bias).

BIBLIOGRAPHY

Chapter 2. Planning a registry. In: Gliklich RE, Dreyer NA, eds. *Registries for Evaluating Patient Outcomes: A User's Guide*. 2nd ed. (Prepared by Outcome DEcIDE Center [Outcome Sciences, Inc. d/b/a Outcome] under contract no. HHSA290200500351 T03.) AHRQ Publication No. 10-EHC049. Rockville, MD: Agency for Healthcare Research and Quality; 2010:23-52.

Bowling A. *Research Methods in Health: Investigating Health and Health Services*. Philadelphia, PA: Open University Press; 1997:163-166.

Sampling

BRIEF DEFINITION

Method of identifying individuals for inclusion in the registry and may include variations such as simple random sampling, stratified sampling, systematic sampling, cluster [area] sampling or multistage sampling.

EXPLANATION

Sampling with a random approach limits systematic bias that may be introduced into the study through the use of nonrandom sampling and is preferred over non-random sampling whenever feasible. Variations of random sampling allow the researcher to select units in which random samples are drawn. Random sampling can be conducted using a systematic approach through computer algorithms from a base population list or as simple as taking every k individual from a list (eg, every 10th person). The important point is that the selection is random and not influenced by the investigator or care team.

VALUE AND USE

The value of the random sample allows for greater generalization of study findings to the base population from which the sample was drawn. For registries and prospective observational studies, random sampling allows a researcher to reduce large sample sizes to manageable numbers for inclusion into the registry.

ISSUES

Random sampling is often difficult because it requires full access to a population which is rarely possible. Most often there is a struggle to obtain enough sample size to meet expectations, rather than having to decrease the sample size. While it is the preferred method of sampling, it is often more difficult to implement and there is often bias introduced as not everyone selected consents to enroll which ultimately biases the randomness of the sampling as the sample is then reduced to those individuals who gave consent to participate (*see term:* Selection Bias).

Random sampling is not always possible and therefore other sampling techniques can be used such as clustering, snowball, stratified and weighted sampling. All of these are less than ideal and represent a nonrandom or convenient sample and care should be taken as to the bias that these sampling techniques introduce into the registry design.

BIBLIOGRAPHY

Bowling A. *Research Methods in Health: Investigating Health and Health Services*. Philadelphia, PA: Open University Press; 1997:163-166.

Chapter 3. Registry design. In: Gliklich RE, Dreyer NA, eds. *Registries for Evaluating Patient Outcomes: A User's Guide*. 2nd ed. (Prepared by Outcome DEcIDE Center [Outcome Sciences, Inc. d/b/a Outcome] under contract no. HHSA290200500351 T03.) AHRQ Publication No. 10-EHC049. Rockville, MD: Agency for Healthcare Research and Quality; 2010:53-78.

Lohr SL. Sampling: Design and Analysis. Boston, MA: Duxbury Press; 1999.

Rothman K, Greenland S. *Modern Epidemiology*. Philadelphia, PA: Lippincott Williams & Wilkins; 1998.

Campbell J. Statistical methods for randomized controlled trials: sample selection bias issues. In: Esposito D, ed. *Reliability and Validity of Data Sources for Outcomes Research & Disease and Health Management Programs*. Lawrenceville, NJ: ISPOR; 2013:421-422.

Comparison Group

BRIEF DEFINITION

A group of patients or participants similar in relevant respects to the intervention or observed study group. They do not receive the intervention or the treatment being principally observed.

EXPLANATION

Registries are usually uncontrolled and therefore do not have a control or comparison group. However, when they do identify a comparison group, it is usually the standard of care or usual care group (*see terms:* Usual Care; Standard of Care). Different ways of incorporating data from comparator groups are discussed below.

» *Internal Comparator*

A subgroup of study patients or participants who are in the same study and similar in relevant respects to the intervention or observed study subgroup. They do NOT receive the intervention, treatment or exposure being principally observed, which in a patient registry is only observed and identified passively.

» *External Comparator*

A group of patients or participants who are not part of the study but are similar in relevant respects to the intervention or observed study group or subgroup. These patients also do not receive the intervention, treatment or exposure being principally observed. For example, the Surveillance Epidemiology and End Results (SEER) cancer registry data can be used as an external comparator for registry studies in cancer.

» *Historical Comparator*

A longitudinal study feature in which an intervention is introduced or observed in a series of participants and the results are compared to the outcome in a previous series of comparable participants.

» *Matched Control*

A participant not receiving the treatment or exposure of interest, but who carries an identical, or nearly identical, profile to a case with regard to all other variables (eg, demographics, risk factors).

VALUE AND USE

Internal comparators allow the analyst to observe differences in outcomes between cohorts under the same general circumstances and timeframe, as these patients are subject to the same set of inclusion/exclusion criteria as the observed study group. By holding many of these otherwise variable features constant, comparative effectiveness and safety inferences, based on a registry's internal comparator, generally carry more internal validity than inferences using alternative comparator types (*see term:* Validity).

In the absence of a valid internal comparator, it would be important to leverage external comparators or historical comparators to provide critical context to help interpret data revealed by a registry.

Matched controls are also very useful in patient registries, as they allow comparators to be simulated while minimizing bias due to differences in baseline characteristics.

ISSUES

It is not feasible to have or sustain a valid internal comparator if there are significantly different characteristics between patients who receive a particular therapy and those who do not, or if there is no reason to maintain a long-term cohort of patients who are not treated with such a therapy.

Furthermore, a major issue with the use of external or historical comparators is that such patients may have different inclusion and/or exclusion criteria and thus, inferences drawn may not be robust and/or invalid.

Regardless of the choice of comparator, it is important to carefully examine the study patients to determine similarity between the groups under comparison. Sensitivity analyses can be used to determine robustness of registry findings, when registry data are analyzed using different comparator groups (*see term:* Sensitivity Analyses).

BIBLIOGRAPHY

Chapter 3. Registry design. In: Gliklich RE, Dreyer NA, eds. Registries for Evaluating Patient Outcomes: A User's Guide. 2nd ed. (Prepared by Outcome DEcIDE Center [Outcome Sciences, Inc. d/b/a Outcome] under contract no. HHSA290200500351 T03.) AHRQ Publication No. 10-EHC049. Rockville, MD: Agency for Healthcare Research and Quality; 2010:53-78.

Rothman K, Greenland S. *Modern Epidemiology.* Philadelphia, PA: Lippincott Williams & Wilkins; 1998.

Mangano DT, Tudor IC, Dietzel C, et al. The risk associated with aprotinin in cardiac surgery. *N Engl J Med.* 2006;354:353-365.

Watson K, Symmons D, Griffiths I, Silman A. The British Society for Rheumatology biologics register. *Ann Rheum Dis.* 2005;64:iv42-iv43.

Duration of Observation

BRIEF DEFINITION

The time interval from inclusion in the registry to the last data entry, which may be either fixed or open-ended.

EXPLANATION

Across all patients in the registry, the duration of observation spans from the baseline observation of the first patient (note that some data could be collected retrospectively) to the last observation of the final patient to be included, should the registry close operations. The duration of observation in patient registries is highly variable, with some registries collecting data at only one time point and others collecting data for the lifetime of the patient. A registry may be open-ended or it may have a fixed end point when enough data to achieve the study objectives is expected to have accrued.

VALUE AND USE

Registries generally require fewer resources and are less burdensome on the participants than interventional studies, and thus are better suited for studying long-term outcomes. Specifying an appropriate duration of observation is essential in ensuring that a study can meet its objectives. For instance, a study designed to measure the incidence of cancer recurrence in patients who received a particular treatment must have a duration of observation that is sufficiently long to allow for the development of the cancer.

ISSUES

Decisions about when to stop a registry are not always straightforward if the registry does not have a predetermined duration of observation. The duration of participant observation in patient registries is usually longer than that of a clinical trial; however, it may be limited to a single episode of care or extend to the lifetime of the patient.

BIBLIOGRAPHY

Rothman KJ, Haas J. When should a patient registry end? Draft white paper for AHRQ patient registries. Handbook II. http://effectivehealthcare.ahrq.gov/repFiles/draftDocuments/2009_0817StoppingARegistry.pdf. Published 2009. Accessed April 24, 2013.

Chapter 2. Planning a registry. In: Gliklich RE, Dreyer NA, eds. *Registries for Evaluating Patient Outcomes: A User's Guide*. 2nd ed. (Prepared by Outcome DEcIDE Center [Outcome Sciences, Inc. d/b/a Outcome] under contract no. HHSA290200500351 T03.) AHRQ Publication No. 10-EHC049. Rockville, MD: Agency for Healthcare Research and Quality; 2010:23-52.

Core Dataset

BRIEF DEFINITION

Set of data variables required to achieve the scientific objectives set out in the protocol.

EXPLANATION

Should be considered as "need to know" and not just "nice to know."

VALUE AND USE

In global (or at least multicountry) registries, data elements comprising the core dataset will appear on the CRFs of all patients in the registry, regardless of country or other defining characteristic.

ISSUES

Balance must be struck between the value of speculative fields and the added burden on sites, patients, and budgets from collecting this information.

BIBLIOGRAPHY

Chapter 2. Planning a registry. In: Gliklich RE, Dreyer NA, eds. *Registries for Evaluating Patient Outcomes: A User's Guide*. 2nd ed. (Prepared by Outcome DEcIDE Center [Outcome Sciences, Inc. d/b/a Outcome] under contract no. HHSA290200500351 T03.) AHRQ Publication No. 10-EHC049. Rockville, MD: Agency for Healthcare Research and Quality; 2010:23-52.

McDevitt J, Comber H. A proposed core national cancer dataset: National Cancer Registry. National Cancer Registry Ireland. http://www.ncri.ie/pubs/pubfiles/CoreNationalCancerDatasetv1.0.pdf. Published December 17, 2009. Accessed April 24, 2013.

Data: Sources, Elements, Capture and Quality Assurance

Primary Data Sources

BRIEF DEFINITION

Data which are collected from individuals to create a registry.

EXPLANATION

Various primary data sources can include all or some of the following individuals:

- **Patients:** provide subjective responses on HRQOL, preferences (utilities), medication use, medication satisfaction, behavioral data, social data, and family history not otherwise attainable by study procedures.
- **Clinicians:** provide useful perceptions on patient clinical impression, diagnosis, and laboratory results. Have access to patients on a regular basis and thus may be able to better describe patient history.
- **Caregivers:** provide unique perceptions of patients and on progression of disease. May also have access to the patient on a regular basis and may assist with recording information in a patient diary.
- **Pharmacists:** provide drug history information including but not limited to adherence, persistence, potential drug interactions, and contraindications.

VALUE AND USE

Primary data collection may increase the probability of completeness, reliability, and validity, based on the measurement and data collection method defined in a registry.

ISSUES

Collecting data from primary data sources is expensive and often has a limited sample size.

BIBLIOGRAPHY

Chapter 6. Data sources for registries. In: Gliklich RE, Dreyer NA, eds. *Registries for Evaluating Patient Outcomes: A User's Guide*. 2nd ed. (Prepared by Outcome DEcIDE Center [Outcome

Sciences, Inc. d/b/a Outcome] under contract no. HHSA290200500351 T03.) AHRQ Publication No. 10-EHC049. Rockville, MD: Agency for Healthcare Research and Quality; 2010:127-141.

Hay J. Statistical approaches and methods. In: Esposito D, ed. *Reliability and Validity of Data Sources for Outcomes Research & Disease and Health Management Programs*. Lawrenceville, NJ: ISPOR; 2013:335-433.

Secondary Data Sources

BRIEF DEFINITION

Previously established sources of patient data.

EXPLANATION

Secondary data sources could include all or some of the following:

» ***Medical Charts***

Provide useful retrospective and prospective information on patient history, current medical condition(s) and outcomes.

» ***Electronic Health Records (EHRs)***

EHRs may be accessed via the hospital or institutional intranet system. They can typically provide real-time data to facilitate more appropriate and timely patient treatment. Many systems are searchable so they can be used to populate a registry with any necessary data.

» ***Institutional or Organizational Databases***

These databases, developed to house patient information, may include reports or audio/visual recordings from diagnostic tests such as X-rays or MRI records. Institutional databases include patients managed or treated at a specified institution. Organizational databases include individuals in a patient organization or other organizations not directly related to a medical institution.

» ***Administrative Databases***

Databases that track patients for billing or coverage purposes which may provide information on resource use.

» ***Birth and Death Records***

Birth records may assist in registries examining pregnancy or birth defects while death records may be used to establish cause of death and whether a patient has been lost to follow-up.

» ***Census Databases***

Contain useful information on the general population and can be used to target the geographical location of a registry or certain populations.

» ***Existing Registries***

Existing or completed registries may be useful in identifying gaps in data that have occurred in previous studies. This information can guide the design of a proposed study so that these deficiencies are eliminated or minimized. Existing registries can also provide contextual information when reporting the new study.

VALUE AND USE

Secondary data sources are useful in some studies for allowing access to existing data; use of secondary data may obviate the need for primary data collection and thereby reduce overall study cost. In addition, secondary sources may provide historical data prior to initiation of prospective data collection, or may be the sole source of data in some studies.

ISSUES

Analyses utilizing secondary data sources are often limited by the type and scope of data available from those sources.

BIBLIOGRAPHY

Berger ML, Mamdani M, Atkins D, Johnson ML. Good research practices for comparative effectiveness research: defining, reporting and interpreting nonrandomized studies of treatment effects using secondary data sources: the ISPOR Good Research Practices for Retrospective Database Analysis Task Force Report—Part I. *Value Health*. 2009;12:1044-1052.

Cox E, Martin BC, Van Staa T, et al. Good research practices for comparative effectiveness research: approaches to mitigate bias and confounding in the design of nonrandomized studies of treatment effects using secondary data sources: the ISPOR Good Research Practices for Retrospective Database Analysis Task Force Report—Part II. *Value Health*. 2009;12: 1053-1061.

Johnson ML, Crown W, Martin BC, et al. Good research practices for comparative effectiveness research: analytic methods to improve causal inference from nonrandomized studies of treatment effects using secondary data sources: the ISPOR Good Research Practices for Retrospective Database Analysis Task Force Report—Part III. *Value Health*. 2009;12: 1062-1073.

Schneeweiss S, Avorn J. A review of uses of health care utilization databases for epidemiologic research on therapeutics. *J Clin Epidemiol.* 2005;58:323-337.

Motheral B, Brooks J, Clark MA, et al. A checklist for retrospective database studies—report of the ISPOR Task Force on Retrospective Databases. *Value Health.* 2003;6:90-97.

Hennessy S. Use of health care databases in pharmacoepidemiology. *Basic Clin Pharmacol Toxicol.* 2006;98:311-313.

Esposito D, ed. *Reliability and Validity of Data Sources for Outcomes Research & Disease and Health Management Programs.* Lawrenceville, NJ: ISPOR; 2013.

Data Domains

BRIEF DEFINITION

A data domain is a collection of data elements that all relate to a common topic.

EXPLANATION

Common data domains in patient registries are exposures, outcomes, and patient demographics. Other domains may be included, depending on the type of study, such as AEs, provider, etc. The Clinical Data Acquisition Standards and Harmonization (CDASH) initiative defines commonly used domains for clinical trials, which may be applied where relevant in registry studies as well. Possible domains include the following:

» ***Exposures***

Data to identify the natural progression of a disease, a condition, a health care service, independent risk factors, and/or procedures.

» ***Outcomes***

The effect on health status from performance (or nonperformance) of one or more processes or activities carried out by health care providers. Health outcomes include morbidity and mortality; physical, social, and mental functioning; nutritional status; and HRQOL. Also categorized as clinical, humanistic, patient reported, economic, as well as intermediate and final. Should include the primary and secondary endpoints of the study (*see term:* Outcomes/End Points).

» ***Patient***

Demographic and other relevant details of the patients who are exposed to the medications and/or criteria applicable to the registry.

» ***Diagnostics***

Identifies patients who have undergone diagnostic tests and the results of those tests.

» ***Provider***

Characteristics of the individuals (typically physicians, but also possibly pharmacists) providing health care interventions to the patients enrolled in the registry.

» ***Environmental***

Environmental factors considered potentially relevant to the exposure of interest in the registry. (For example, exposure to asbestos or environmental factors such as behaviors, air/noise pollution, cleanliness (sterility), patient contact in hospitals, patient room interactions, etc.)

» ***Adverse Events***

Data on all AEs occurring during the course of the registry, including timing, relatedness to a product of interest, and severity (*see term:* Safety).

VALUE AND USE

Domains are useful for the organization of data collection and analysis. Establishing domains and elements within domains helps to ensure concise and logical data collection.

ISSUES

Although domain-based data collection is usually implemented, for some longitudinal registries, a visit-based data structure is used instead.

BIBLIOGRAPHY

Clinical Data Interchange Standards Consortium. Clinical Data Acquisition Standards and Harmonization (CDASH). http://www.cdisc.org/stuff/contentmgr/files/0/9b32bc345908ac4c31ce72b529a3d995/misc/cdash_std_1_0_2008_10_01.pdf. Published October 1, 2008. Accessed December 20, 2010.

Chapter 5. Data elements for registries. In: Gliklich RE, Dreyer NA, eds. *Registries for Evaluating Patient Outcomes: A User's Guide*. 2nd ed. (Prepared by Outcome DEcIDE Center [Outcome Sciences, Inc. d/b/a Outcome] under contract no. HHSA290200500351 T03.) AHRQ Publication No. 10-EHC049. Rockville, MD: Agency for Healthcare Research and Quality; 2010:103-125.

Data Definitions

BRIEF DEFINITION

Defines pertinent registry parameters including exposures/treatments, tests, and outcomes.

EXPLANATION

Data elements should be defined in such a way that researchers are able to consistently report data in the same manner as one another, and from one time point to the next (measurement reliability). Valid ranges and values for each element should be clearly stated. Data definitions can also include the logical relationship of elements to one another.

VALUE AND USE

Clear and precise data definitions are critical for ensuring the internal validity of the study (*see term:* Validity).

ISSUES

Using published clinical data standards for data elements, if available, is preferred as it allows for greater comparability between studies and makes data linkage efforts more feasible. Clinical data standards for some diseases/outcomes have been published and are widely agreed upon (eg, cancer, cardiology); other diseases lack such standards.

BIBLIOGRAPHY

Chapter 5. Data elements for registries. In: Gliklich RE, Dreyer NA, eds. *Registries for Evaluating Patient Outcomes: A User's Guide*. 2nd ed. (Prepared by Outcome DEcIDE Center [Outcome Sciences, Inc. d/b/a Outcome] under contract no. HHSA290200500351 T03.) AHRQ Publication No. 10-EHC049. Rockville, MD: Agency for Healthcare Research and Quality; 2010:103-125.

Cannon CP, Battler A, Brindis RG, et al. American College of Cardiology key data elements and definitions for measuring the clinical management and outcomes of patients with acute coronary syndromes: a report of the American College of Cardiology Task Force on Clinical Data Standards (Acute Coronary Syndromes Writing Committee). *J Am Coll Cardiol*. 2001;38:2114–2130.

McNamara RL, Brass LM, Drozda JP Jr, et al. ACC/AHA key data elements and definitions for measuring the clinical management and outcomes of patients with atrial fibrillation: a report of the American College of Cardiology/American Heart Association Task Force on Clinical Data Standards (Writing Committee to Develop Data Standards on Atrial Fibrillation). *Circulation*. 2004;109:3223–3243.

Radford MJ, Arnold JM, Bennett SJ, et al. ACC/AHA key data elements and definitions for measuring the clinical management and outcomes of patients with chronic heart failure: a report of the American College of Cardiology/American Heart Association Task Force on Clinical Data Standards (Writing Committee to Develop Heart Failure Clinical Data Standards): developed in collaboration with the American College of Chest Physicians and the International Society for Heart and Lung Transplantation: endorsed by the Heart Failure Society of America. *Circulation*. 2005;112:1888–1916.

Data Capture/Collection

BRIEF DEFINITION

The recording and collecting of study data at the site through patient/participant examinations, laboratory determinations, interviews, questionnaires, patient charts, electronic medical records, hospital records, and death certificates.

EXPLANATION

As prospective studies, typically with collection of at least some data that may not have been captured in routine practice, patient registries should conform to clinical data guidelines similar to those which apply to interventional trials (*see term:* Ethics and Privacy).

VALUE AND USE

The collection methods, if developed to be comprehensive and easily completed by site staff, can be useful tools to ensure that the study operates efficiently and on schedule while also reducing missing data and other potential sources of bias due to investigator error. Collection methods can take multiple forms including web-based electronic or paper charts. Other methods include scanning techniques for uploading of documents.

ISSUES

The collection methods typically require significant consideration and field testing to ensure that they are comprehensive, fully represent the Statistical Analysis Plan (SAP) or protocol and are understandable by the site staff (*see term:* Analysis Plan).

BIBLIOGRAPHY

Bowling A. *Research Methods in Health: Investigating Health and Health Services*. Philadelphia, PA: Open University Press; 1997:163-166.

Chapter 10. Data collection and quality assurance. In: Gliklich RE, Dreyer NA, eds. *Registries for Evaluating Patient Outcomes: A User's Guide*. 2nd ed. (Prepared by Outcome DEcIDE Center [Outcome Sciences, Inc. d/b/a Outcome] under contract no. HHSA290200500351 T03.) AHRQ Publication No. 10-EHC049. Rockville, MD: Agency for Healthcare Research and Quality; 2010:225-252.

Instrument or Scale Validation

BRIEF DEFINITION

The psychometric and statistical validation of a PRO instrument prior to its use in the registry, or the adaptation of a given PRO scale to a slightly different population than it was originally intended for.

EXPLANATION

Psychometric assessment includes a series of analysis looking at validity, reliability, responsiveness, and clinical meaningfulness (See below for descriptions).

» ***Content Validity***

The association between the content of a measurement instrument and the domain of knowledge it purports to represent. Content validity tests that the instrument is measuring the concept it is intended to measure. Qualitative studies such as patient interviews, focus groups, and cognitive interviews are used to generate items and to provide evidence that the items and domains are appropriate and comprehensive. Content validity is the first measurement property that must be verified; if content validity is not demonstrated then testing other measurement properties is useless.

» ***Construct Validity***

The degree to which the relationship between items and domains follows the hypothesized conceptual framework.

» ***Criterion Validity***

The degree to which instrument scores are related to a criterion measure. A criterion measure is a standard, external measure that measures a similar concept to that of the instrument being validated. Criterion validity often cannot be measured for PROs due to a lack of accepted measures in this field of study.

» ***Reliability***

The degree to which an instrument is free from random error, usually defined in terms of internal consistency and reproducibility. Internal consistency describes a situation in which all items that contribute to a scale are measuring the same concept. Internal consistency is measured using Cronbach's alpha for summary scores and item-total correlations. Reproducibility measures whether the score is stable when the instrument is administered at different time points or by different interviewers and there is no change expected in the concept being measured; these are often referred to as test-retest, intra-interviewer, and inter-interviewer reliability. This provides evidence that any differences between subjects or changes in scores over time are the result of true differences or changes in what the scale purports to measure, and not due to factors related to instrument administration.

» ***Responsiveness***

The extent to which an instrument measures change over time. A PRO instrument, for example, should be able to distinguish changes in scores over time in subjects who have changed with respect to the concept being measured.

» ***Interpretability/Clinical Meaningfulness***

Scores and changes in score can be interpreted according to a meaningful clinical framework. Validation of a PRO should include guidance on how particular scores should be interpreted in relation to the clinical outcome of interest. An attempt should be made to ascertain clinically meaningful benchmarks for different score levels (*see term:* Health-Related Quality of Life [HRQOL] Outcomes).

VALUE AND USE

Because PRO tools measure the subjective patient experience, it is important to confirm that they consistently measure what they claim to measure. Validation of the tool prior to use helps ensure that the results will be valid, reliable, and interpretable.

ISSUES

Creating and validating a new PRO instrument is a time-consuming, iterative process. Before work begins on creating a new tool, a thorough review of available tools should be conducted to verify that there is not already an existing tool that could be used or modified for use.

BIBLIOGRAPHY

U.S. Department of Health and Human Services FDA Center for Drug Evaluation and Research; U.S. Department of Health and Human Services FDA Center for Biologics Evaluation and Research; U.S. Department of Health and Human Services FDA Center for Devices and Radiological Health. Guidance for industry: patient-reported outcome measures: use in medical product development to support labeling claims: draft guidance. *Health Qual Life Outcomes.* 2006;4:79.

Frost MH, Reeve BB, Liepa AM, et al. What is sufficient evidence for the reliability and validity of patient-reported outcome measures? *Value Health.* 2007;10:S94-S105.

Assessing health status and quality-of-life instruments: attributes and review criteria. *Qual Life Res.* 2002;11:193-205.

Fayers PM, Machin D. *Quality of Life: Assessment, Analysis, and Interpretation.* West Sussex, UK: John Wiley & Sons Ltd; 2000.

Messick S. Validity. In: Linn RL, ed. *Educational Measurement.* 3rd ed. National Council on Measurement in Education and American Council on Education, Series in Higher Education. Phoenix, AZ: Oryx Press; 1993.

Messick S. Validity of psychological assessment: validation of inferences from persons' responses and performances as scientific inquiry into score meaning. *Am Psychol.* 1995;50:741-749.

Pedhazur EJ, Schmelkin LP. *Measurement, Design and Analysis: An Integrated Approach.* Hillsdale, NJ: Lawrence Erlbaum Associates; 1991.

Streiner DL, Norman GR. *Health Measurement Scales: A Practical Guide to Their Development and Use*. 2nd ed. New York, NY: Oxford University Press; 1995.

Esposito D, ed. *Reliability and Validity of Data Sources for Outcomes Research & Disease and Health Management Programs*. Lawrenceville, NJ: ISPOR; 2013.

Rothman M, Burke L, Erickson P, et al. Use of existing patient-reported outcome (PRO) instruments and their modification: the ISPOR good research practices for evaluating and documenting content validity for the use of existing instruments and their modification: PRO Task Force Report. *Value Health*. 2009;12:1075-1083.

Patrick DL, Burke LB, Gwaltney CJ, et al. Content validity: establishing and reporting the evidence in newly-developed patient-reported outcomes (PRO) instruments for medical product evaluation: ISPOR PRO Good Research Practices Task Force report: Part 1—eliciting concepts for a new PRO instrument. *Value Health*. 2011;14:967-977.

Patrick DL, Burke LB, Gwaltney CJ, et al. Content validity: establishing and reporting the evidence in newly-developed patient-reported outcomes (PRO) instruments for medical product evaluation: ISPOR PRO Good Research Practices Task Force report: Part 2—assessing respondent understanding. *Value Health*. 2011;14:978-988.

Case Report Forms (CRFs)

BRIEF DEFINITION

The formatted listing of data elements that can be presented in paper or electronic format to facilitate data collection in a patient registry.

EXPLANATION

CRFs dictate the information to be obtained from various data collection sources; the completeness and accuracy of the data acquired will determine the scope of data that will be available for analysis to support the results of the study.

VALUE AND USE

The CRF provides a roadmap for sites to input data throughout the data collection process. These collection tools provide a systematic approach to collection. Standardization to ensure limited errors and missing data are the goals.

ISSUES

CRFs in patient registries need to be relatively simple and easy to complete. In some studies, however, forms can be cumbersome and lengthy, requiring many inputs and resulting in fields that are sometimes left incomplete. Translations in multinational trials sometimes overlook dialect issues and interpretation. Wording, if vague, can leave the site staff to make decisions about data input that are not systematic and introduce random error within the measures.

BIBLIOGRAPHY

Friedman LM, Furberg CD, DeMets DL. *Fundamentals of Clinical Trials*. 4th ed. New York, NY: Springer; 2010:204.

Chapter 10. Data collection and quality assurance. In: Gliklich RE, Dreyer NA, eds. *Registries for Evaluating Patient Outcomes: A User's Guide*. 2nd ed. (Prepared by Outcome DEcIDE Center [Outcome Sciences, Inc. d/b/a Outcome] under contract no. HHSA290200500351 T03.) AHRQ Publication No. 10-EHC049. Rockville, MD: Agency for Healthcare Research and Quality; 2010:225-252.

Mode of Administration

BRIEF DEFINITION

This is the method by which data collection is achieved, eg, written questionnaire, telephone interview, direct clinician report, web based, interactive voice response formats, and combination of the above methods.

EXPLANATION

Clinical and survey data in a registry can be collected using CRFs and questionnaires, which can be administered via a traditional paper route or using electronic data capture (EDC). In evaluating the mode of administration, it is important to consider subject burden, recall bias, interviewer bias, subject's willingness to disclose sensitive information, and secondary data entry errors.

VALUE AND USE

Multimode data collection approaches can be used to increase sample representativeness and response rate, and reduce the amount of missing data. However, there is a great deal of risk to comparability of data when mixing modes of administration.

ISSUES

Registries commonly employ tools that facilitate data collection (ie, web-based, telephone and other EDC options which may be more subject-friendly). As in clinical trial designs, registries should avoid as many sources of error variance in the data as possible. Measurement error can be introduced into a study design by different data capture modes that are not providing comparable data (ie, the modes lack sufficient measurement equivalence.) Measurement error reduces statistical power and attenuates the ability of the study to detect real change (ie, treatment effect) in the end point. Measurement equivalence of questionnaires when using different modes of administration is critical to ensure quality of data collection and comparability of resulting data.

BIBLIOGRAPHY

U.S. Food and Drug Administration. Guidance for industry: patient-reported outcome measures: use in medical product development to support labeling claims. http://www.fda.gov/downloads/Drugs/GuidanceComplianceRegulatoryInformation/Guidances/UCM193282.pdf. Published December 2009. Accessed April 24, 2013.

Bowling A. Mode of questionnaire administration can have serious effects on data quality. *J Public Health*. 2005;27:281-291.

Coons SJ, Gwaltney CJ, Hays RD, et al. Recommendations on evidence needed to support measurement equivalence between electronic and paper-based patient-reported outcome (PRO) measures: ISPOR ePRO Good Research Practices Task Force Report. *Value Health*. 2009;12: 419-429.

Eremenco SE, Coons SJ, Paty J, et al. Mixing modes of patient-reported outcomes data collection in clinical trials: Report of the ISPOR PRO Good Research Practices Task Force Report. *Value Health*. 2013; In press. Available from: http://www.ispor.org/workpaper/practices_index.asp.

Electronic Data Capture

BRIEF DEFINITION

The recording and collecting of study data at the site and directly from the patient, by way of mobile devices, desktop and laptop computers, or by telephone. Examples of the latter include interactive voice response system (IVRS), or text messaging.

EXPLANATION

Technological advances have created many more options for transportable, real-time data entry in both clinical trials and prospective registries. Together, these computer- or device-based methods are commonly referred to as EDC.

VALUE AND USE

EDC methods facilitate data collection, particularly directly from patients, but must be subject to security, privacy, and change control procedures. Flexible formats mean that data capture is available outside of traditional clinical settings. The ease of copying, storing, and repurposing electronic data brings along with it increased risk of inappropriate use.

ISSUES

Care should be taken to ensure that electronic sources are accessible at the sites. As previously discussed, paper as a mode of administration should not be used with EDC (*see term:* Mode of Administration).

BIBLIOGRAPHY

Association for Clinical Data Management (ACDM). Computer systems validation in clinical research: A practical guide (Edition 2). http://www.acdm.org.uk/resources.aspx. Published 2004. Accessed April 24, 2013.

European Medicines Agency (EMA). Reflection paper on expectations for electronic source data and data transcribed to electronic data collection tools in clinical trials. http://www.ema.europa.eu/docs/en_GB/document_library/Regulatory_and_procedural_guideline/2010/08/WC500095754.pdf. Published June 9, 2010. Accessed April 24, 2013.

U.S. Food and Drug Administration. Guidance for industry. Computerized systems used in clinical investigations. http://www.fda.gov/downloads/Drugs/GuidanceComplianceRegulatoryInformation/Guidances/UCM070266.pdf. Published May 2007. Accessed April 24, 2013.

Bowling A. Mode of questionnaire administration can have serious effects on data quality. *J Public Health*. 2005;27:281-291.

Coons SJ, Gwaltney CJ, Hays RD, et al. Recommendations on evidence needed to support measurement equivalence between electronic and paper-based patient-reported outcome (PRO) measures: ISPOR ePRO Good Research Practices Task Force Report. *Value Health*. 2009;12: 419-429.

Eremenco SE, Coons SJ, Paty J, et al. Mixing modes of patient-reported outcomes data collection in clinical trials: Report of the ISPOR PRO Good Research Practices Task Force Report. *Value Health*. 2013; In press. http://www.ispor.org/workpaper/practices_index.asp. Accessed April 24, 2013.

Database Build

BRIEF DEFINITION

The process by which the system is developed for capturing, processing, and exporting the registry data in order to maintain its accuracy, completeness and structural integrity.

EXPLANATION

Registry data is often collected over a long span of time and by personnel at multiple sites. A well-planned central database is critical for maintaining data integrity. Consistency and standardization across multiple users can be improved by incorporating edit checks into the initial database build. Applicable clinical data standards for the relevant setting should be researched and implemented during database design (*see terms:* Edit Checks/Specifications; Clinical Data Standards).

VALUE AND USE

Documentation on the database build with specific instructions, road maps and editing logs provide an invaluable resource for future analysis as well as other activities that incorporate the database such as augmentation, historical comparisons or regulatory requirements.

ISSUES

The database build can become very complex and technical which can make it difficult to understand for researchers outside the immediate user group. Care should be taken during the database build to ensure a broad audience of users for documentation and clearly defined structure and detail in its conception.

BIBLIOGRAPHY

Hummel J. Building a computerized disease registry for chronic illness management of diabetes. *Clin Diab*. 2000;18:107.

Chapter 10. Data collection and quality assurance. In: Gliklich RE, Dreyer NA, eds. *Registries for Evaluating Patient Outcomes: A User's Guide*. 2nd ed. (Prepared by Outcome DEcIDE Center [Outcome Sciences, Inc. d/b/a Outcome] under contract no. HHSA290200500351 T03.) AHRQ Publication No. 10-EHC049. Rockville, MD: Agency for Healthcare Research and Quality; 2010:225-252.

Clinical Data Standards

BRIEF DEFINITION

Standardized approach to collecting data in a registry, generally consisting of standardized data elements with corresponding formats and definitions.

EXPLANATION

Clinical data standards have been promulgated to make comparison, data linkages, and analysis easier across different data sources. These standards are relevant to both EDC and database design for traditional paper-based CRFs.

VALUE AND USE

Compliance with clinical data standards ensures standardization across data sources ultimately providing more robust data from which to evaluate the population.

ISSUES

While these standards propose to ensure standardization across different data sources, not all organizations or registry objectives may be addressed and as a result, individual attention through SOPs may be needed.

BIBLIOGRAPHY

Clinical Data Interchange Standards Consortium, Electronic Source Data Interchange (eSDI) Group. Leveraging the CDISC standards to facilitate the use of electronic source data within clinical trials. Version I. http://www.cdisc.org/stuff/contentmgr/files/0/2f6eca8f0df7caac5bbd4fadfd76d575/miscdocs/esdi.pdf. Published November 20, 2006. Accessed April 24, 2013.

Health Level Seven International (HL7). http://www.hl7.org/. Accessed April 24, 2013.

International Organization for Standardization (ISO). http://www.iso.org/iso/home.html. Accessed April 24, 2013.

Data Quality Assurance

BRIEF DEFINITION

A process of affirming that the data were collected in accordance with established procedures and that they meet the requisite standards of quality to accomplish the registry's intended purposes and the intended use of the data.

EXPLANATION

Key points in ensuring data quality include the advanced publishing of information about the project, developing a study plan/protocol containing the scientific objectives, establishing a sample size justification and a description of the planned analyses, and the timely publishing of a summary of the results after completion of the study. The quality of the data can be improved by using standardized CRFs, and the CRFs should be reviewed and pilot tested before initiation of the full study (*see term:* Case Report Forms). Some measure of source-data verification should be performed in randomly selected centers. Edit checks and data cleaning are steps taken to ensure quality and accuracy of the dataset (*see terms:* Edit Checks/Specifications; Data Cleaning).

A statistical analysis plan (SAP) should be created before initiating statistical analyses (*see terms:* Analysis Plan; STROBE). The use of standardized tables and figures is highly recommended. The basis of the report writing should be the STROBE statement *Strengthening the Reporting of Observational Studies in Epidemiology Initiative* containing a checklist of 22 points to be covered in the report. The development of specific SOPs, describing the processes during planning, conduct and evaluation of a noninterventional study, as well as the quality management and the regular training of all involved personnel, is also highly recommended. However, all accompanying measures to improve or maintain the quality of the patient registry should not compromise the observational nature of the registry.

VALUE AND USE

Quality checks can prove pivotal in ensuring that the data are of a high quality and accurately reflect the protocol; however, while this process is required, it can also be time consuming. The value of these quality assurance tasks is that they ensure the data are as free of error as possible, and that they are implemented to reduce systematic and random bias introduced into the study.

ISSUES

A risk-based approach in developing a quality assurance plan is recommended based on identifying the most important or likely sources of error or potential lapses in procedures that may impact the quality of the registry and the ability to evaluate the primary objective. Regularly applied processes can highlight strengths and weaknesses in data collection. Reporting the results of these audits, including error rates and data completeness, is important for use of the data and interpretation of registry findings.

BIBLIOGRAPHY

Theobald K, Capan M, Herbold M, et al. Quality assurance in non-interventional studies. *Ger Med Sci.* 2009;7:Doc29.

Meling T, Harboe K, Arthursson AJ, Søreide K. Steppingstones to the implementation of an inhospital fracture and dislocation registry using the AO/OTA classification: compliance, completeness and commitment. *Scand J Trauma Resusc Emerg Med.* 2010;18:54.

Thoburn KK, German RR, Lewis M, et al. Case completeness and data accuracy in the Centers for Disease Control and Prevention's National Program of Cancer Registries. *Cancer.* 2007;109:1607-1616.

Edit Checks/Specifications

BRIEF DEFINITION

Rules applied to database entries to ensure logic and consistency throughout the database.

EXPLANATION

Edit checks and field specifications are built in to data capture and/or data entry systems at the time of design. Rules may include restrictions on data type and format (eg, numeric; structured text choices), data range (eg, eligible dates, ages), and data completion (required fields). In contrast to these *a priori* quality checks, data cleaning will generally take place on the completed dataset prior to locking the data for analysis (*see term:* Data Cleaning).

VALUE AND USE

Edit checks and field specifications reduce common errors that may be missed during data input and limit biases associated with data input that may plague further activities within the study.

ISSUES

Edit checks and field specifications are time-consuming operations and need to be budgeted accordingly, both in time and budget. Care should be taken to provide systematic approaches to incorporating these activities throughout the data input process and conformity to standards is necessary.

BIBLIOGRAPHY

Chapter 10. Data collection and quality assurance. In: Gliklich RE, Dreyer NA, eds. *Registries for Evaluating Patient Outcomes: A User's Guide.* 2nd ed. (Prepared by Outcome DEcIDE Center [Outcome Sciences, Inc. d/b/a Outcome] under contract no. HHSA290200500351 T03.) AHRQ

Publication No. 10-EHC049. Rockville, MD: Agency for Healthcare Research and Quality; 2010:225-252.

CDISC Clinical Research Glossary, v 8.0. http://www.cdisc.org/stuff/contentmgr/files/0/be-650811feb46f381f0af41ca40ade2e/misc/cdisc_2009_glossary.pdf. Published December 2009. Accessed April 24, 2013.

Data Cleaning

BRIEF DEFINITION

The correction or minimization of data problems in the live database, including missing values, incorrect or out-of-range values, or logically inconsistent responses (*see term:* Missing Observations).

EXPLANATION

Data-cleaning efforts for registry data should be directed toward the most important areas, those most crucial to answering the primary study question.

VALUE AND USE

Data cleaning is facilitated by EDC, as the programmed edit checks clean data in real time and data managers do not need to wait for paper forms to be processed (*see term:* Electronic Data Capture).

ISSUES

Observational data can present challenges for data cleaning since procedures, available data and expected values may not be standard across the participating sites.

BIBLIOGRAPHY

Van den Broeck J, Cunningham SA, Eeckels R, Herbst K. Data cleaning: detecting, diagnosing, and editing data abnormalities. *PLoS Med.* 2005;2:e267.

Pomerantseva V. What every data manager should know about clinical trial data. Pharmapro.com. http://www.pharmpro.com/Articles/2009/04/Clinical-DataCleaning-and-Validation-Steps/. Published April 15, 2009. Accessed April 24, 2013.

On-site Monitoring

BRIEF DEFINITION

Regular observation and recording of activities taking place at registry sites, to inform and improve study performance and outputs.

EXPLANATION

Monitoring activities are common in clinical trials and other studies that need to conform to the 21 Code of Federal Regulations (*see term:* US Food and Drug

Administration [FDA] Regulations). Sometimes patient registries also need to conform to these and other regulations and, as such, monitoring activities may be implemented in these studies. Monitoring typically includes an evaluation of the study's data accuracy or integrity, as well as the site's compliance with the study protocol and procedures. If performed on-site, some or all registry data are generally compared with source data from medical records, and sites can also be assessed for their overall compliance with study procedures. On-site monitoring normally occurs less frequently—or not at all—in observational studies compared to RCTs.

VALUE AND USE

Monitoring plays an important role in ensuring the quality of registry processes and data; it helps validate data points and creates a record for these checks and verifications. Training of clinical research associates (CRAs) in on-site monitoring activities is rigorous and formalized through various organizations such as the Society for Clinical Research Associates (SoCRA) and the Association of Clinical Research Professionals (ACRP) (*see term:* Clinical Research Associate). Both are excellent sources for more information.

ISSUES

Inconsistencies between CRFs and source documentation indicate error and potentially abuse. Additionally, on-site monitoring may generate a Hawthorne effect, where the behavior of the site may potentially be altered because it knows it is being observed and monitored in-person, as opposed to remotely, or not at all. This awareness that the site will be monitored generally enhances diligent data recording.

BIBLIOGRAPHY

The Society of Clinical Research Associates (SoCRA). http://www.socra.org/. Accessed April 24, 2013.

Association of Clinical Research Professionals (ACRP). http://www.acrpnet.org/. Accessed April 24, 2013.

Food and Drug Administration. Guidance for industry oversight of clinical investigations: a risk-based approach to monitoring. 2011: 6-8. http://www.fda.gov/downloads/drugs/guidancecomplianceregulatoryinformation/guidances/ucm269919.pdf. Accessed April 24, 2013.

Centralized or Remote Monitoring

BRIEF DEFINITION

Clinical monitoring that does not involve CRAs or site-management associates visiting registry sites, but is most often conducted via telephone.

EXPLANATION

Observational research does not typically include—or require—the same level of, or approach to, monitoring seen in interventional trials. In most registries, a remote and low-frequency-monitoring approach is seen as adequate and appropriate; this approach is less financially burdensome on the study budget and on the sites, while providing an important quality assurance review of study data and performance. Monitoring typically includes an evaluation of the study's data accuracy or integrity, as well as the site's compliance with the study protocol and procedures.

VALUE AND USE

These relaxed monitoring activities reduce unnecessary costs, while ensuring some monitoring and data validation.

ISSUES

Centralized/Remote monitoring may not be appropriate for all protocols, such as those requiring intervention, conformance with the 21 Code of Federal Regulations, or other regulatory approaches (*see term:* US Food and Drug Administration [FDA] Regulations).

BIBLIOGRAPHY

Food and Drug Administration. Guidance for industry oversight of clinical investigations: a risk-based approach to monitoring. 2011: 6-8. http://www.fda.gov/downloads/drugs/guidancecomplianceregulatoryinformation/guidances/ucm269919.pdf. Accessed April 24, 2013.

Site Support and Data Management

Site Identification and Recruitment

BRIEF DEFINITION

The means by which registry sites are identified for participation. The process usually involves providing to sites, under a confidentiality agreement, a protocol synopsis and a brief questionnaire that evaluates the site's interest and capabilities.

EXPLANATION

Site selection for observational studies/registries typically seeks to represent a particular population, such as the general prescribing population, community-based practices only, or prescribers for a particular indication. In addition, sites may be identified in a way that achieves balance by site/investigator characteristics including geography, practice size and prescription frequency (ie, high- and low-volume prescribers). Sites may be research-naïve and, following initial identification, are assessed to ensure that they can comply with any requirements to participate.

VALUE AND USE

Similar to patient recruitment and selection, the methodology for targeting particular sites and investigators is a critical determinant of the representativeness of any findings from the registry; this is especially true of observational research that includes elements of physician behavior such as treatment patterns and adherence to guidelines. Identifying the appropriate sites, capable of recruiting patients and complying with study processes, is also critical in achieving study objectives. A registry will usually have a large number of sites, and efforts to identify high-quality sites at the start of the study will support efficient patient recruitment, data collection, and query resolution efforts throughout the study. Registries often involve many research-naïve and community-based sites, offering an opportunity to evaluate real-world care; these sites, however, may find it much more challenging to meet the requirements of the study and to follow key operational steps.

ISSUES

Even if the methodology for choosing sites for recruitment is well established and documented, some bias may be introduced by the pattern of sites that choose to participate. In addition to not offering patients a treatment free of charge, the inability of registries and other observational studies to provide adequate monetary compensation can be a deciding factor for otherwise-qualified sites.

BIBLIOGRAPHY

Chapter 9. Recruiting and retaining participants in the registry. In: Gliklich RE, Dreyer NA, eds. *Registries for Evaluating Patient Outcomes: A User's Guide.* 2nd ed. (Prepared by Outcome DEcIDE Center [Outcome Sciences, Inc. d/b/a Outcome] under contract no. HHSA290200500351 T03.) AHRQ Publication No. 10-EHC049. Rockville, MD: Agency for Healthcare Research and Quality; 2010:207-223.

Site Start-up

BRIEF DEFINITION

The processes required to prepare a site for patient enrollment and data collection in a registry.

EXPLANATION

Site start-up is a critical step in the conduct of a registry and constitutes a range of tasks, depending on the registry design, that may be performed on-site or remotely. For large registries with limited and relatively simple data collection, start-up may be streamlined. The site start-up process includes obtaining any required and completed regulatory documents from the site, negotiating a contract and budget, supporting IRB or IEC submissions (either via a local or central IRB) and training site staff (*see term:* Institutional Review Board [IRB]/Ethical Committee Approval).

VALUE AND USE

From a regulatory standpoint, the site start-up is critical in ensuring each site's ability to perform the study, and to ensure that key documents are in place prior to any patient enrollment. Sites are the primary vehicle for recruiting and retaining patients and obtaining clinical and outcomes data.

ISSUES

If not effectively managed, the site start-up process can be prolonged, and can significantly affect the registry's ability to meet enrollment milestones. For sites, especially those that are research naïve, the start-up period represents an important reinforcement of the requirements for participation (eg, AE reporting, IRB responsibilities, ability to conduct EDC), and sets the stage for their participation throughout the study.

BIBLIOGRAPHY

Chapter 9. Recruiting and retaining participants. In: Gliklich RE, Dreyer NA, eds. *Registries for Evaluating Patient Outcomes: A User's Guide*. 2nd ed. (Prepared by Outcome DEcIDE Center [Outcome Sciences, Inc. d/b/a Outcome] under contract no. HHSA290200500351 T03.) AHRQ Publication No. 10-EHC049. Rockville, MD: Agency for Healthcare Research and Quality; 2010:207-223.

Site Training

BRIEF DEFINITION

The process by which sites are educated regarding registry/study procedures and data collection requirements, including use of EDC systems.

EXPLANATION

A critical step to ensure that sites are properly prepared and that the study has a good chance of succeeding.

VALUE AND USE

Site training is conducted with all sites and is designed to educate the physician and study staff that will be supporting the registry, on the study procedures. This training includes reviewing the registry protocol, patient eligibility criteria, patient enrollment and follow-up procedures, safety-event reporting (either via a data collection process within the study or through normal reporting requirements (eg, MedWatch) [*see term:* Safety]), patient discontinuation processes, and study close-out procedures. Sites and staff should also be trained on any additional study tools, such as EDC systems and administration of any patient HRQOL questionnaires (*see terms:* Electronic Data Capture; Health-Related Quality of Life [HRQOL] Outcomes). Training is a critical step in ensuring that sites are properly prepared to complete all study tasks so that each will submit high-quality data in a timely manner.

ISSUES

Documentation of site training does not exonerate investigators or project management staff of wrongdoings or errors made. It simply acts as a systematic process to help ensure that the protocol and data collection instruments are communicated and understood. Ongoing training should occur over the course of the study to address issues not foreseen at study start-up.

BIBLIOGRAPHY

Chapter 9. Recruiting and retaining participants. In: Gliklich RE, Dreyer NA, eds. *Registries for Evaluating Patient Outcomes: A User's Guide*. 2nd ed. (Prepared by Outcome DEcIDE Center [Outcome Sciences, Inc. d/b/a Outcome] under contract no. HHSA290200500351 T03.) AHRQ Publication No. 10-EHC049. Rockville, MD: Agency for Healthcare Research and Quality; 2010:207-223.

Regulatory Documents

BRIEF DEFINITION

Required documents that allow a site to participate in a registry and enroll patients. Examples include investigator curriculum vitae (CV), copy of medical license and signed contract with sponsor/ARO/CRO and, when applicable, IRB approval.

EXPLANATION

As is the case with all clinical trials, key documents must be executed prior to enrolling patients. At a minimum, sites must have a signed contract that documents their responsibilities and requirements for participating in the study. In addition to the contract, in studies where patients will be enrolled and followed, confirmation of IRB/IEC approval will be required.

VALUE AND USE

Since registries look at real-world clinical settings, the risk-benefit profile must be considered when determining what documentation is required.

ISSUES

Regulatory documentation varies by regulating body even though there are several international guidelines such as those stated above. Care should be taken to seek out appropriate regulatory bodies of each governing nation or region in which the registry is being established (*see term:* Ethics and Privacy). In addition, documentation must be put in perspective of the research conducted (postmarketing registry versus phase III trial) as many requirements may not apply in a noninterventional setting.

BIBLIOGRAPHY

Chapter 2. Planning a registry. In: Gliklich RE, Dreyer NA, eds. *Registries for Evaluating Patient Outcomes: A User's Guide*. 2nd ed. (Prepared by Outcome DEcIDE Center [Outcome Sciences, Inc. d/b/a Outcome] under contract no. HHSA290200500351 T03.) AHRQ Publication No. 10-EHC049. Rockville, MD: Agency for Healthcare Research and Quality; 2010:23-52.

Investigator Meetings

BRIEF DEFINITION

Meetings, conducted either in person or via webcast, where participating physicians/investigators and/or site personnel are trained on the protocol and registry procedures.

EXPLANATION

These meetings typically include training sessions for investigators and staff that promote standardization of procedures, and help to minimize error during the course of the study; training should cover operational processes and technical measurements. This meeting may be led, in part, by a registry's SAB members (*see term:* Scientific Advisory Board [SAB]).

VALUE AND USE

Although less commonly used in registries than in RCTs, investigator meetings can provide an opportunity to motivate sites, encourage enrollment, and share interim results (if permitted by the analysis plan). Investigator meetings for registries may be considered optional compared to the effort required for RCT participation, are more likely to be performed remotely (eg, via webinar) and may be regional or targeted to areas where the impact may be greatest. Often, multiple online meetings are scheduled to accommodate prolonged site-enrollment schedules and sites' time zones and schedules. Investigator meetings can be an effective tool for helping establish a registry community and for supporting communication and best practices among sites.

ISSUES

In some cases, the sheer number of participating sites in a registry precludes comprehensive investigator meetings. Care must be taken when conducting investigator meetings in the setting of observational studies and registries that routine clinical practice is not affected by participation.

BIBLIOGRAPHY

Chapter 2. Planning a registry. In: Gliklich RE, Dreyer NA, eds. *Registries for Evaluating Patient Outcomes: A User's Guide.* 2nd ed. (Prepared by Outcome DEcIDE Center [Outcome Sciences, Inc. d/b/a Outcome] under contract no. HHSA290200500351 T03.) AHRQ Publication No. 10-EHC049. Rockville, MD: Agency for Healthcare Research and Quality; 2010:23-52.

Patient Recruitment

BRIEF DEFINITION

The process of enrolling patients into the study.

EXPLANATION

Patients may be recruited via a variety of methods, including through recruited sites/investigators or directly. In most cases, the physician (or site staff) will provide the patient with details of the registry, requirements for participation (which are usually minimal, as patients are treated and followed per standard of care), and the informed consent form (or assent form in cases where the registry participant is a minor (*see terms:* Informed Consent; Recruitment and Retention Tools)).

VALUE AND USE

Efficient and well-documented patient recruitment, coupled with patient retention, supports the analytic objectives of the study, and is perhaps the most important determinant of registry success. As with site/investigator recruitment, the methodology of patient recruitment is critical to understanding the resultant patient population and interpretation of any results. Understanding the population from which the study population was drawn is integral to establishing the external validity of the results drawn from the study (*see term:* Validity).

ISSUES

The rate of patient recruitment, whether predicted by the sponsor, advisory boards, investigators or other stakeholders, invariably will need to be adjusted once the registry is actually initiated. Competition from ongoing clinical trials and other observational studies, changes in routine practice and other aspects of the real world all may contribute to slow or inconsistent recruitment, and recruitment strategies may need to be adjusted accordingly.

BIBLIOGRAPHY

Anderson D. *A Guide to Patient Recruitment and Retention.* Boston, MA: CenterWatch; 2004.

Chapter 9. Recruiting and retaining participants in the registry. In: Gliklich RE, Dreyer NA, eds. *Registries for Evaluating Patient Outcomes: A User's Guide.* 2nd ed. (Prepared by Outcome DEcIDE Center [Outcome Sciences, Inc. d/b/a Outcome] under contract no. HHSA290200500351 T03.) AHRQ Publication No. 10-EHC049. Rockville, MD: Agency for Healthcare Research and Quality; 2010:207-223.

Patient Retention

BRIEF DEFINITION

Maintaining patient participation throughout the study is often a challenge in long-term observational studies where the benefit to the patient may be modest or low.

EXPLANATION

Multiple factors can affect patient-retention rates including the length of follow-up, the data collection requirements, and patient transfers from registry enrolling sites to unenrolled providers.

VALUE AND USE

Patient-retention rates affect the analytical power. Furthermore, if systematic differences in rates of participation exist between study groups (often referred to as nonresponse or participation bias), then study validity can be questioned. Plans to improve retention such as increased patient outreach, or patient incentives (for instance access to treatment results included in the registry reports) should be defined and budgeted for during registry design. Similarly, contingency plans to obtain data for patients lost to follow-up (such as linkage to existing data sources), if possible, should be defined to minimize the impact of nonresponse bias.

ISSUES

Efforts to increase patient retention may impose selection bias (*see term:* Selection Bias). It is important to consistently adhere to predefined inclusion and exclusion criteria and enrollment strategies.

BIBLIOGRAPHY

Chapter 9. Recruiting and retaining participants in the registry. In: Gliklich RE, Dreyer NA, eds. *Registries for Evaluating Patient Outcomes: A User's Guide*. 2nd ed. (Prepared by Outcome DEcIDE Center [Outcome Sciences, Inc. d/b/a Outcome] under contract no. HHSA290200500351 T03.) AHRQ Publication No. 10-EHC049. Rockville, MD: Agency for Healthcare Research and Quality; 2010:207-223.

Newberry A, Sherwood P, Hricik A, et al. Understanding recruitment and retention in neurological research. *J Neurosci Nurs*. 2010;42:47-57.

Recruitment and Retention Tools

BRIEF DEFINITION

Methods used to promote awareness of the registry/study and encourage continued participation by sites/investigators and patients.

EXPLANATION

Since reimbursement levels for registries are typically much lower than the compensation for participating in RCTs, recruitment and motivational tools are often important for both site recruitment and patient retention. Recruitment tools may include direct physician and/or patient outreach. Strategies include actively searching for participants by identifying target groups (by reviewing hospital admissions, searching records, or setting up a testing facility), directly inviting study participants (by advertising through mass media, leaflets, or health fairs), and approaching third parties for assistance (by physician letters, telephone calls, presentations at professional society meetings, notices in professional journals, or exhibits at scientific conferences). Additional approaches may be used to motivate sites and retain patients, such as creating a community among participants, providing informational resources (such as study newsletters and patient education materials), and providing publication opportunities to investigators.

VALUE AND USE

Recruitment and retention tools can help encourage sites to both initially participate and then continue to provide quality data throughout the duration of the registry.

ISSUES

Efforts to increase enrollment and retention of study participants may impose selection bias (for instance targeting high-volume or academic-based practices or centers).

BIBLIOGRAPHY

Chapter 9. Recruiting and retaining participants in the registry. In: Gliklich RE, Dreyer NA, eds. *Registries for Evaluating Patient Outcomes: A User's Guide*. 2nd ed. (Prepared by Outcome DEcIDE Center [Outcome Sciences, Inc. d/b/a Outcome] under contract no. HHSA290200500351 T03.) AHRQ Publication No. 10-EHC049. Rockville, MD: Agency for Healthcare Research and Quality; 2010:207-223.

Newberry A, Sherwood P, Hricik A, et al. Understanding recruitment and retention in neurological research. *J Neurosci Nurs*. 2010;42:47-57.

Site Reimbursement

BRIEF DEFINITION

Monetary payments made from the registry sponsor to investigator sites, commensurate with the level of effort required by the protocol (usually significantly less than that involved in RCTs) and the number of patients enrolled at that site.

EXPLANATION

Sites may be reimbursed for their start-up costs and time spent recording data. They are not paid directly for recruiting or enrolling patients.

VALUE AND USE

Reimbursement for fair-market value of the effort required to participate in the registry is a motivation for participation, and may provide important support at the site for staff, especially at sites where specific research resources do not exist.

ISSUES

The required or requested rate of reimbursement may differ from site to site, and can be affected by hospital or other institutional requirements. Reimbursement must be consistent with the fair market value of time spent, which can be estimated by pilot testing the CRF. If site payment is considerably higher than that commensurate with the level of effort required by the protocol, then the sponsor runs the risk of not being in compliance with the Anti-Kickback Statute.

BIBLIOGRAPHY

Lader EW, Cannon CP, Ohman EM, et al. The clinician as investigator: participating in clinical trials in the practice setting. *Circulation*. 2004;109:2672-2679.

Office of Inspector General. Office of Public Affairs. Federal Anti-Kickback Law and Regulatory Safe Harbors: Fact Sheet. http://oig.hhs.gov/fraud/docs/safeharborregulations/safefs.htm. Published November 1999. Accessed April 24, 2013.

Patient Honoraria

BRIEF DEFINITION

Compensation made to study participants, commensurate with level of effort required by the registry protocol.

EXPLANATION

Compensation (eg, store or currency gift cards, registry-branded materials such as calendars and notepads) may be provided to patients, generally as a token of appreciation for the patient's completion of particular milestones.

VALUE AND USE

Patient honoraria can be a useful motivational tool, particularly when the study involves PROs and longer periods of follow-up.

ISSUES

Patient compensation, whether monetary or nonmonetary, is not always acceptable (ie, may be considered an inducement by ethics committees) and its use may depend on the regions/countries where the registry is being conducted.

BIBLIOGRAPHY

Chapter 9. Recruiting and retaining participants in the registry. In: Gliklich RE, Dreyer NA, eds. *Registries for Evaluating Patient Outcomes: A User's Guide*. 2nd ed. (Prepared by Outcome DEcIDE Center [Outcome Sciences, Inc. d/b/a Outcome] under contract no. HHSA290200500351 T03.) AHRQ Publication No. 10-EHC049. Rockville, MD: Agency for Healthcare Research and Quality; 2010:207-223.

Grady C, Dickert N, Jawetz T, et al. An analysis of U.S. practices of paying research participants. *Contemp Clin Trials*. 2005;26:365-375.

Loss to Follow-up

BRIEF DEFINITION

Patients who are no longer available for follow-up and who no longer respond to outreach attempts (by the site or study staff) to determine their status.

EXPLANATION

Over the course of a registry or study, some patients may be lost to follow-up where their status and reason for discontinuation are unknown. Soliciting the contact information of patient's next of kin or other secondary contact can help mitigate this problem. It is important to note that loss to follow-up (also referred to as attrition) does not imply the end of treatment; although these individuals are not able to be studied further, they may or may not have continued with the treatment of interest.

VALUE AND USE

This term is used to characterize patients for whom intended duration of follow-up was not achieved and the reason for discontinuation is not known.

ISSUES

Loss to follow-up can be problematic if it occurs frequently and nonrandomly. If the reason for discontinuation is unknown, there is the possibility that the patients remaining in the registry are systematically different in important ways from the patients that were lost. In addition, the patient may have discontinued participation due to an outcome of interest. Differential rates in loss to follow-up or attrition for subjects with a particular exposure or disease can impose bias (follow-up or attrition bias) which can substantially affect the conclusions and interpretation of results (*see terms:* Missing Observations; Strategies for Handling Missing Observations). If possible, contingency plans to obtain data for patients lost to follow-up (such as linkage to existing data sources) should be defined. Follow-up rates or other measures of attrition (such as the relative risk of dropping out or of stopping the intervention, or factors predicting loss to follow-up) should be reported since substantial and nonrandom attrition can jeopardize the validity of research findings.

BIBLIOGRAPHY

Chapter 9. Recruiting and retaining participants in the registry. In: Gliklich RE, Dreyer NA, eds. *Registries for Evaluating Patient Outcomes: A User's Guide*. 2nd ed. (Prepared by Outcome DEcIDE Center [Outcome Sciences, Inc. d/b/a Outcome] under contract no. HHSA290200500351 T03.) AHRQ Publication No. 10-EHC049. Rockville, MD: Agency for Healthcare Research and Quality; 2010:207-223.

Hunt JR, White E. Retaining and tracking cohort study members. *Epidemiol Rev.* 1998;20:57-70.

Krishnan E, Murtagh K, Bruce B, et al. Attrition bias in rheumatoid arthritis databanks: a case study of 6346 patients in 11 databanks and 65,649 administrations of the Health Assessment Questionnaire. *J Rheumatol.* 2004;31:1320-1326.

Eysenbach G. The law of attrition. *J Med Internet Res.* 2005;7:e11.

Enrollment Log/Screening Log

BRIEF DEFINITION

A tool used to track which eligible patients are enrolled in the registry/study and which are not, and why patients were designated as such.

EXPLANATION

Unlike RCTs, in registries true screening processes or testing is not typically performed. If consecutive eligible patient enrollment is desired, however, enrollment logs are often requested to better understand those who ended up in the registry and those who did not. When used, the enrollment/screening log is a tool (either via paper or online via the study EDC system) for tracking all patients that are approached for recruitment in a registry. The log will include patients that are both enrolled and not enrolled. Typically for patients enrolled, the log will note the unique patient number; for patients not enrolled, the reason for nonparticipation will be documented. In summary, the patient enrollment/screening log provides documentation of all individuals who are evaluated for participation in a registry/research study. Further, it provides information on study progress of all enrolled patients and on early withdrawals/termination of patients (*see term:* Patient Recruitment).

VALUE AND USE

A screening log provides critical information for characterizing the enrolled patient population, assessing the potential for selection bias, and determining future recruitment efforts.

ISSUES

While highly useful in theory, the validity of these logs, in practice, may be limited. In the absence of some way of randomly auditing these logs via medical record or billing record review, their accuracy may be questionable. For example, completion of enrollment logs may be considered cumbersome by sites, decreasing their accuracy as a measure of patient screening and enrollment.

BIBLIOGRAPHY

National Institute of Neurological Disorders. National Institutes of Health. NINDS glossary of clinical research terms. http://www.ninds.nih.gov/research/clinical_research/basics/glossary.htm. Updated February 10, 2010. Accessed April 24, 2013.

Barsness G, Feldman AM, Holmes DR, et al. The International EECP Patient Registry (IEPR): design, methods, baseline characteristics, and acute results. *Clin Cardiol.* 2001;24:435-442.

Performance Measure

BRIEF DEFINITION

A metric used to gauge study progress, such as site or patient enrollment (eg, patients per site per month) and CRF completion status.

EXPLANATION

A tool that may be used by the sponsor, site, CRA or other registry staff to track progress. These metrics are centered on a site's performance, which may include patient recruitment and follow-up, completeness of data, and completed patients.

VALUE AND USE

For the sponsor/CRO, these performance measures allow the tracking of enrollment rates and, if using EDC, the rate of CRF completion. These measures allow, in real time, identification of sites that may be underperforming, require retraining, or may need to be closed out.

ISSUES

Sites, as well as sponsors, may be interested in benchmarking performance compared to projections and/or to other sites. However, site details and investigator-specific information may be considered sensitive or confidential. For this reason, typically each site may have access to view only their own progress in detail, and may also be able to see their performance in comparison with aggregated measures from other sites. Explicit project management activities should be employed here to gauge progress of the registry. Specific measures should be drafted and evaluated throughout the process, with built in quality checks.

BIBLIOGRAPHY

Chapter 9: Recruiting and retaining participants in the registry. In: Gliklich RE, Dreyer NA, eds. *Registries for Evaluating Patient Outcomes: A User's Guide*. 2nd ed. (Prepared by Outcome DEcIDE Center [Outcome Sciences, Inc. d/b/a Outcome] under contract no. HHSA290200500351 T03.) AHRQ Publication No. 10-EHC049. Rockville, MD: Agency for Healthcare Research and Quality; 2010:207-223.

Help Desk

BRIEF DEFINITION

Telephone/Email support provided by study operations staff to sites for answers to study questions. The scope of help desk support depends on the nature of the study and the capabilities of the help desk (eg, limited to technical questions regarding the EDC system, addressing IRB interaction documentation issues etc.).

EXPLANATION

The help desk supports sites by responding to study questions, whether they are related to the study protocol, data entry (either on paper-based CRFs or online via EDC), request for study supplies, or other issues related to the site's participation in the registry. The help desk can often be reached by telephone, email, or a study website portal. Regional help desk support (with relevant language capabilities) may also mitigate site frustration or loss of interest and can help with transition of site personnel, which is common in long-term registries and at sites without dedicated research staff.

VALUE AND USE

The help desk is an essential component in ensuring site questions are answered in a timely manner and enhances ongoing participation in the registry. It is particularly important in studies involving EDC, as the ability to quickly get assistance with username/password changes, data entry issues and other nonclinical issues may be resolved without involvement of a CRA (*see terms:* Electronic Data Capture; Case Report Forms).

ISSUES

The help desk does not take the place of CRAs or other registry-related staff, and roles should be clearly delineated to avoid site confusion

BIBLIOGRAPHY

Chapter 10: Data collection and quality assurance. In: Gliklich RE, Dreyer NA, eds. *Registries for Evaluating Patient Outcomes: A User's Guide*. 2nd ed. (Prepared by Outcome DEcIDE Center [Outcome Sciences, Inc. d/b/a Outcome] under contract no. HHSA290200500351 T03.) AHRQ Publication No. 10-EHC049. Rockville, MD: Agency for Healthcare Research and Quality; 2010:225-252.

Clinical Research Associate (CRA)

BRIEF DEFINITION

Person who oversees the progress and conduct of the registry/study to ensure the quality of data collected, to monitor the progress of study enrollment and progress, and to serve as a primary contact for the site. This individual may also be referred to as a study coordinator or site manager.

EXPLANATION

The role of the CRA in registries versus RCTs may be quite different. In both cases, the CRA is the main point of contact for the site and their participation in the registry, including ongoing communication with the site, remote site management, and query resolution. In registries however, regular onsite data monitoring and complete source data verification, typical roles for the CRA in an RCT, are usually restricted to risk-based or random-sampling method monitoring.

VALUE AND USE

Local CRAs are often the best source of information regarding country-specific regulations, issues surrounding site recruitment and contracting and local standard practices, all of which can be critical to efficient start-up.

ISSUES

Communication lines between CRAs in the field and centralized CRAs and other registry staff must be well established in order to identify potential data collection and other site issues as soon as possible. For postmarketing registries, the role of local medical science liaisons (and similar sponsor personnel) versus the role of CRAs should be determined *a priori* in order to avoid any potential issues affecting relationships with the sites.

BIBLIOGRAPHY

The Society of Clinical Research Associates (SoCRA). http://www.socra.org/. Accessed April 24, 2013.

Association of Clinical Research Professionals (ACRP). http://www.acrpnet.org/. Accessed April 24, 2013.

Food and Drug Administration. Guidance for industry oversight of clinical investigations: a risk-based approach to monitoring. 2011: 6-8. http://www.fda.gov/downloads/drugs/guidancecomplianceregulatoryinformation/guidances/ucm269919.pdf. Accessed April 24, 2013.

Source Document Verification (SDV)

BRIEF DEFINITION

SDV is the process by which the study staff confirms that accurate and reliable information has been reported by the investigator to the sponsor during the study and is a fundamental requirement of good clinical practice (GCP) (*see term:* Evaluating and Ensuring Registry Quality).

EXPLANATION

SDV is generally performed as a part of monitoring by comparing the data provided to the registry (either the CRFs or the database itself) with the source documentation at the site, which may include medical records, laboratory results or paper PRO forms. The level of SDV for registries should reflect the key analytic variables and the data identified as potentially at risk for inaccuracies.

VALUE AND USE

In registries, 100% SDV is rarely conducted, nor is it required. Rather, SDV may be performed on a random sample of study sites or of data fields within sites, often at a lower frequency, such as 10% of sites throughout the study.

ISSUES

In the case of EDC-based studies, source data, such as PROs, may be entered directly into the database without a paper source; therefore, true SDV is sometimes not possible and data quality must rely on edit and form controls. If errors are found via SDV, it is unclear what level of data incompleteness or variation in quality among sites is acceptable.

BIBLIOGRAPHY

Chapter 10. Data collection and quality assurance. In: Gliklich RE, Dreyer NA, eds. *Registries for Evaluating Patient Outcomes: A User's Guide*. 2nd ed. (Prepared by Outcome DEcIDE Center [Outcome Sciences, Inc. d/b/a Outcome] under contract no. HHSA290200500351 T03.) AHRQ Publication No. 10-EHC049. Rockville, MD: Agency for Healthcare Research and Quality; 2010:225-252.

Nahm ML, Pieper CF, Cunningham MM. Quantifying data quality for clinical trials using electronic data capture. *PLoS One*. 2008;3:e3049.

Rostami R, Nahm M, Pieper CF. What can we learn from a decade of database audits? The Duke Clinical Research Institute experience, 1997-2006. *Clin Trials*. 2009;6:141–150.

Query Resolution

BRIEF DEFINITION

Query resolution involves contacting the source of specific data (eg, a specific site) to address an incomplete or invalid response on the CRF, or other assessment completed by the site. Queries are usually triggered by automatic edit checks built into the database, but may also arise from manual data quality checks.

EXPLANATION

Queries are generally only made of the sites. Patient reported responses are rarely, if ever, queried.

VALUE AND USE

Queries are a standard data management tool to maximize the completeness and quality of the data.

ISSUES

Queries, if they become extensive and numerous, can be very burdensome to many registry sites. Queries should be limited to data elements deemed key or critical.

BIBLIOGRAPHY

Chapter 10. Data collection and quality assurance. In: Gliklich RE, Dreyer NA, eds. *Registries for Evaluating Patient Outcomes: A User's Guide*. 2nd ed. (Prepared by Outcome DEcIDE Center [Outcome Sciences, Inc. d/b/a Outcome] under contract no. HHSA290200500351 T03.) AHRQ Publication No. 10-EHC049. Rockville, MD: Agency for Healthcare Research and Quality; 2010.

Close-out

Site Close-out

BRIEF DEFINITION

The steps taken by the study monitoring staff to formally complete all transactions and communication with the investigative sites.

EXPLANATION

Site close-out procedures are often in the form of a checklist and may include activities such as ensuring that all data analyses and sponsor queries, remaining administrative tasks (such as IRB final progress reports and final enrollment logs), and financial accounting have been completed.

VALUE AND USE

Site close-out procedures ensure the timely and accurate submission of all required reports and adjustments for amounts due.

ISSUES

Site close-out procedures should also ensure that data privacy is maintained even after patient recruitment is complete to protect against potential abuses of the privacy of patient's health information (*see term:* Record Retention and Database Archiving).

BIBLIOGRAPHY

The HMO Research Network. Multi-site Closeout Guide. http://www.researchtoolkit.org/primer/docs/HMORN_Closeout%20Guide.pdf. Published October 11, 2006. Accessed April 24, 2013.

Dinnett EM, Mungall MB, Kent JA, et al. Closing out a large clinical trial: lessons from the prospective study of pravastin in the elderly at risk (PROSPER). *Clin Trials.* 2004;1:545-552.

Data Transfer

BRIEF DEFINITION

The exchange of raw data from the study database, or analytic datasets from the ARO or CRO, to the study sponsor.

EXPLANATION
Policies for data transfer may be outlined as part of site close-out SOPs.

VALUE AND USE
Transfer of the raw patient data or analytic datasets may be needed by the study sponsor for publication of study data or future research.

ISSUES
Data transfer is typically conditional on data ownership and is something that should be clearly defined during the registry planning and development stages (*see term:* Stakeholders).

BIBLIOGRAPHY
Chapter 2. Planning a registry. In: Gliklich RE, Dreyer NA, eds. *Registries for Evaluating Patient Outcomes: A User's Guide*. 2nd ed. (Prepared by Outcome DEcIDE Center [Outcome Sciences, Inc. d/b/a Outcome] under contract no. HHSA290200500351 T03.) AHRQ Publication No. 10-EHC049. Rockville, MD: Agency for Healthcare Research and Quality; 2010:23-52.

Record Retention and Database Archiving

BRIEF DEFINITION
The manner and duration of study documentation and database storage. Study documents typically include the protocol and any amendments, the SAP, completed CRF and diary pages, site visit documentation, study timetables, flow charts and planned vs. actual enrollment, etc. Electronic study database storage should include steps taken to ensure security of the data (eg, password protection [*see term:* Data Protection]).

EXPLANATION
At a minimum, the study archive should contain, or refer to, the following:

- Study protocol and all approved modifications;
- A final report of the study;
- All source data and, where feasible, any biologic specimens retained in normal clinical practice. A printed sample of the master computer data file(s), if feasible, with reference to the location of the machine-readable master. All source data should comprise the raw data that provided the basis for the final analysis of the study. The archival material should be sufficiently detailed to permit re-editing and re-analysis;
- Adequate documentation to allow identification and location of all computer programs and statistical procedures used, including version numbers where appropriate;

- Copies of electronic versions of analytic datasets and programs, computer printouts, if feasible, including relevant execution codes, which form the basis of any tables, graphs, discussions, or interpretations in the final report. Any manually developed calculations should be documented on a work sheet and similarly retained;
- Correspondence pertaining to the study, SOPs, informed consent releases, copies of all relevant representative material, copies of signed IRB and other external reviewer reports, and copies of all quality assurance reports and audits;
- Communication of study results to the sponsor, regulators, and scientific community should be documented, including, for example; questionnaires; name, make and model numbers of relevant measurement instruments; calibration information and procedures;
- Documentation relating to the collection and processing of study data, including laboratory/research notebooks, training and reference documents for abstracts, interviews, and coders.

VALUE AND USE

Complete and detailed record retention and database archiving are essential for the support of future publication and additional research, if applicable. Complete records also are essential for verifying the quality of study data produced and demonstrating investigator compliance with GCP guidelines and applicable regulatory requirements.

ISSUES

Policies surrounding what records to store and duration of storage can vary across research organizations, although storage and archiving rules for particular types of data may be subject to relevant state and federal laws.

BIBLIOGRAPHY

National Institutes of Health. Office of the Director. Guidelines for the Conduct of Research in the Intramural Research Program at NIH. http://sourcebook.od.nih.gov/ethic-conduct/Conduct%20 Research%206-11-07.pdf. Published May 2007. Accessed April 24, 2013.

Evaluating and Ensuring Registry Quality

Agency for Healthcare Research and Quality Guidance for Registries

BRIEF DEFINITION

Methods to ensure registry quality have been defined in a handbook produced by the Agency of Healthcare Research and Quality in the US (first edition published in 2007 and a second in 2010). This document provides guidance on the creation, operation and evaluation of registries used to assess patient outcomes.

EXPLANATION

It has a US focus, providing basic information on key areas of registry development and operations, highlighting the spectrum of practices in each of these areas and their potential strengths and weaknesses, and is illustrated with case examples. It also provides a practical guide to the day-to-day operational issues and decisions for producing and interpreting high-quality registries. A section on evaluation summarizes key points to facilitate review of the structure, data, and interpretations of patient registries, describing good registry practice in terms of basic elements and potential enhancements. A third edition is in development.

VALUE AND USE

The aim of this publication is to help researchers establish, manage, and analyze patient registries to evaluate the real-life impact of health care treatments and evaluate patient outcomes. Importantly, the content reflects the perspectives and experience of numerous contributors, and represents the current state of understanding in patient registry design, management, and analysis.

ISSUES

Like any publication, this handbook does not address every potential question in this important methodology. When seeking guidance in a patient registry, it is important to consider this reference along with other available guidelines and standards, particularly when addressing issues in global programs or ex-US challenges.

BIBLIOGRAPHY

Chapter 10: Data collection and quality assurance. In: Gliklich RE, Dreyer NA, eds. *Registries for Evaluating Patient Outcomes: A User's Guide*. 2nd ed. (Prepared by Outcome DEcIDE Center [Outcome Sciences, Inc. d/b/a Outcome] under contract no. HHSA290200500351 T03.) AHRQ Publication No. 10-EHC049. Rockville, MD: Agency for Healthcare Research and Quality; 2010:225-252.

European Medicines Agency's (EMA) Guidance on HRQOL

BRIEF DEFINITION

In the drug approval context, HRQOL is considered a specific type of PRO.

EXPLANATION

The guidance defines a PRO as "any outcome directly evaluated by the patient and based on patient's perception of a disease and its treatment(s)." EMA uses PRO as an umbrella term encompassing both single and multidimension domains; that is, measures of symptoms, health status, and satisfaction with treatment. HRQOL is one of these multidimensional assessments under the PRO heading, broadly defined as a patient's subjective perception of the effects of the disease and treatment(s) on daily life, well-being, and psychological, physical, and social functioning. It is clearly differentiated from core symptoms of a disease (*see term:* Health-Related Quality of Life [HRQOL] Outcomes).

VALUE AND USE

This guidance discusses the place that HRQOL may have in the drug evaluation process and gives some broad recommendations on its use in the context of already existing guidance documents. These recommendations are relevant to a variety of study designs including registry-based HRQOL assessments.

BIBLIOGRAPHY

European Medicines Agency. Reflection Paper on the Regulatory Guidance for the Use of Health Related Quality of Life (HRQL) Measures in the Evaluation of Medicinal Products. http://www.ispor.org/workpaper/emeahrql-guidance.pdf. Published July 2005. Accessed April 24, 2013.

European Network of Centres for Pharmacoepidemiology and Pharmacovigilance (ENCePP)

BRIEF DEFINITION

An organization affiliated with the EMA designed to further strengthen the post-authorization monitoring of European medicinal products throughout their lifecycle by facilitating the conduct of multicenter, independent, postauthorization studies focusing on safety and benefit/risk ratio.

EXPLANATION

ENCePP is a key initiative within the European Risk Management Strategy (ERMS) led by the EMA. ENCePP's Code of Conduct provides a set of principles for conducting pharmacoepidemiology and pharmacovigilance studies. Electronic registries and health care databases are included. It complements existing legislation and associated rules and guidelines, but does not replace existing relevant legislation (eg, Directive 2001/20/EC in the case of clinical trials).

VALUE AND USE

The ENCePP Database of Research Resources provides a searchable electronic index of the available EU pharmacoepidemiology and pharmacovigilance research resources. These resources include research centers and networks as well as a registry of EU pharmacoepidemiological and pharmacovigilance studies.

BIBLIOGRAPHY

ENCePP. http://www.encepp.eu. Updated April 22, 2013. Accessed April 24, 2013.

Guidelines for Good Pharmacoepidemiology Practices (GPP)

BRIEF DEFINITION

These guidelines are produced by the International Society for Pharmacoepidemiology (ISPE) and are intended to assist investigators with issues pertaining to the planning, conduct and evaluation of pharmacoepidemiologic research, which can include data from registries.

EXPLANATION

The first revision in 2004 revised and superseded the Guidelines for Good Epidemiologic Practice (GEP) developed in 1996. In that revision, the scope of the guidelines was broadened geographically and conceptually to include risk management and pharmacoeconomic activities and to address more clearly the role of epidemiologic studies from industry and regulatory perspectives so as to reflect ISPE's international membership. Specifically it provided guidance on regulatory reporting requirements as they relate both to individual cases and to aggregate data. The focus of the second revision is on the use and communication of statistical measures and to add clarification to specific items throughout the document.

VALUE AND USE

The ISPE GPP Guidelines propose minimum practices and procedures that should be considered to help ensure the quality and integrity of pharmacoepidemiologic research, and to provide adequate documentation of research methods and results. Pharmacoepidemiology is the core science of risk assessment and the evaluation of the effectiveness of risk-minimization interventions. As such, the GPP also support risk-management activities.

It should be noted that regulatory guidance supersedes those of societies and accrediting bodies. The guidance for industry from the FDA serves as a role model for appropriate conduct in accordance with the expectations of the US regulatory authority. Other national regulatory agencies should be consulted as variation in international guidance may persist.

ISSUES

There has been inconsistent adoption of these guidelines among regulatory bodies, so care should be taken to ensure regulatory compliance first and then these guidelines provide a roadmap for appropriate pharmacoepidemiologic practices.

BIBLIOGRAPHY

Epstein P. Guidelines for good pharmacoepidemiology practices (GPP). *Pharmacoepidemiol Drug Saf.* 2005;14:589-595.

International Society for Pharmacoepidemiology. Guidelines for Good Pharmacoepidemiology Practices (GPP). http://www.pharmacoepi.org/resources/guidelines_08027.cfm. Updated April 2007. Accessed April 24, 2013.

Guidance for Industry: Good Pharmacovigilance Practices and Pharmacoepidemiological Assessment

BRIEF DEFINITION

These guidelines have been developed by the US Department of Health and Human Services. They provide guidance on good pharmacovigilance practices and pharmacoepidemiologic assessment of observational data regarding drugs, including biological drug products but excluding blood and blood components. The guidelines specifically address safety-signal identification, pharmacoepidemiologic assessment and safety-signal interpretation, as well as the development of pharmacovigilance plans.

EXPLANATION

The guidelines give recommendations on how to achieve effective, efficient, consistent, and valid pharmacovigilance practices, with accurate assessment on the nature and level of a drug reaction. Although the guidance was developed by the

US Department of Health and Human Services, the framework for good pharmacovigilance process is not limited to US circumstances.

VALUE AND USE

Regulatory guidance supersedes those of societies and accrediting bodies. As noted above, the guidance for industry from the FDA serves as a role model for appropriate conduct in accordance with the expectations of the US regulatory authority. Other national regulatory agencies should be consulted as there may be variation in international guidance.

BIBLIOGRAPHY

Final guidance: good pharmacovigilance practices and pharmacoepidemiologic assessment. *Biotechnology Law Rep.* 2005;24:344-356.

U.S. Department of Health and Human Services, Food and Drug Administration. Guidance for Industry: Good Pharmacovigilance Practices and Pharmacoepidemiologic Assessment. http://www.fda.gov/downloads/RegulatoryInformation/Guidances/UCM126834.pdf. Published March 2005. Accessed April 24, 2013.

Guidelines for Evaluating Public Health Surveillance Systems

BRIEF DEFINITION

These guidelines, prepared by the Centers for Disease Control, describe tasks and related activities that can be applied to registries when used as a public health surveillance system.

EXPLANATION

Public health surveillance is the ongoing, systematic collection, analysis, interpretation, and dissemination of data about a health-related event for use in planning public health action to reduce morbidity and mortality and to improve health. Areas of particular relevance include establishment of data standards and the electronic exchange of health data.

VALUE AND USE

The guidelines provide information on how to assess the quality of surveillance systems. They address a wide audience, including public health practitioners; health care providers; data providers and users; professional, private, and nonprofit organizations; and government officials at the local, state, and federal levels.

BIBLIOGRAPHY

Centers for Disease Control and Prevention. Updated guidelines for evaluating public health surveillance systems. Recommendations from the guidelines working group. *MMWR Recomm Rep*. 2001;50(RR13):1-35.

Publication of updated guidelines for evaluating public health surveillance systems. *JAMA*. 2001;286:1446.

Swedish Association of the Pharmaceutical Industry (LIF): Rules for Noninterventional Studies

BRIEF DEFINITION

These rules set out the criteria for pharmaceutical companies' participation in the performance of noninterventional studies.

EXPLANATION

Noninterventional studies include all studies and projects which are not classified as clinical trials, according to the Swedish Medical Products Agency. These rules include quality projects, follow-up studies, prescription studies, etc. The rules also apply to participation in, or support for, the establishment or operation of various registries.

The rules were developed by the Swedish Association of the Pharmaceutical Industry, but could also be generalized to other areas. They regulate the principles for prescription of a drug in relation to the decision to include the patient in the registry, the manner in which the drug should be prescribed, and ethical rules for financial compensation to health care providers when enrolling a patient in a registry.

VALUE AND USE

The rules for noninterventional studies form part of the Ethical Rules for the Pharmaceutical Industry in Sweden. These rules apply to collaboration of pharmaceutical companies with the public and private healthcare sector for noninterventional studies.

BIBLIOGRAPHY

The Swedish Association of the Pharmaceutical Industry (LIF). Ethical rules for the pharmaceutical industry in Sweden. http://www.lif.se/default.aspx?id=52392. Updated June 30, 2010. Accessed April 24, 2013.

Good Research Practice Considerations

CONSORT (Consolidated Standard of Reporting Trials)

BRIEF DEFINITION

The CONSORT statement provides specifications for reporting RCTs and its extensions, such as pragmatic trials.

EXPLANATION

The CONSORT statement was derived to improve reporting of RCTs and focuses on minimizing the risk of bias (internal validity). The original CONSORT statement has been updated and revised with recommendations on reporting of AEs in clinical trials and on reporting of noninferiority and equivalence trials. In addition, one of the extensions of the CONSORT statement was derived to improve the reporting of pragmatic trials and is focused on applicability in a range of usual care settings. Application of CONSORT appears to have improved the quality of reporting of trials. The most up-to-date revision of the CONSORT Statement is CONSORT 2010 and details regarding the CONSORT statement and its extensions can be accessed from the website: http://www.consort-statement.org/consort-statement/overview0/.

The CONSORT specifications include a checklist of 25 items related to effective reporting of clinical trial data. The checklist was developed because empirical evidence indicates that failure to report trial information in a transparent manner leads to biased estimates of treatment effects and because the information is essential to judge the reliability or relevance of the findings.

The 25-item checklist for CONSORT specifications is presented in the following categories:

- Title and abstract;
- Introduction: background and objectives;
- Methods: trial design, changes to trial design, participants, study settings, interventions, outcomes, changes to outcomes, sample size, interim analyses and stopping guidelines, randomization-sequence generation, randomization type, randomization-allocation concealment mechanism, randomization implementation, blinding (masking), similarity of interventions, statistical methods, additional analyses;

- Results: participant flow, losses and exclusion, recruitment, reason for stopped trial, baseline data, numbers analyzed, outcomes and estimation, binary outcomes, ancillary analyses, harms;
- Discussion: limitations, generalizability, interpretation;
- Other information: registration, protocol, funding.

Further, the CONSORT group has announced that a new extension for reporting QOL data from clinical trials is under development.

VALUE AND USE

The CONSORT statement enables readers to understand a trial's design, conduct, analysis and interpretation, and to assess the validity of its results. However, this can only be achieved through complete transparency from authors. Although designed for RCTs, some of the elements in CONSORT are relevant to the reporting of registries.

ISSUES

Not all items of the CONSORT recommended guidelines are applicable to patient registries. In addition, the CONSORT statement does not provide detailed information on safety evaluations.

BIBLIOGRAPHY

CONSORT. Transparent Reporting of Trials. http://www.consort-statement.org/. Accessed April 24, 2013.

Schulz KF, Altman DG, Moher D; CONSORT Group. CONSORT 2010 Statement: updated guidelines for reporting parallel group randomised trials. *Ann Int Med.* 2010;152:726-732.

Ioannidis JP, Evans SJ, Gotzsche PC, et al. Better reporting of harms in randomized trials: an extension of the CONSORT statement. *Ann Intern Med.* 2004;141:781-788.

Piaggio G, Elbourne DR, Altman DG, et al. Reporting of noninferiority and equivalence randomized trials: an extension of the CONSORT statement. *JAMA.* 2006;295:1152-1160.

Altman DG, Schulz KF, Moher D, et al. The revised CONSORT statement for reporting randomized trials: explanation and elaboration. *Ann Intern Med.* 2001;134:663-694.

Moher D, Jones A, Lepage L; CONSORT Group (Consolidated Standards for Reporting of Trials). Use of the CONSORT statement and quality of reports of randomized trials: a comparative before-and-after evaluation. *JAMA.* 2001:285:1992-1995.

Plint AC, Moher D, Morrison A, et al. Does the CONSORT checklist improve the quality of reports of randomised controlled trials? A systematic review. *Med J Aust.* 2006;185:263-267.

Husereau D, Drummond M, Petrou S, et al. Consolidated Health Economic Evaluation Reporting Standards (CHEERS)—Explanation and Elaboration: A Report of the ISPOR Health Economic Evaluations Publication Guidelines Good Reporting Practices Task Force. *Value Health.* 2013;16:231-250.

GRACE (Good ReseArch for Comparative Effectiveness)

BRIEF DEFINITION

The GRACE Checklist is designed for the assessment of observational studies of comparative effectiveness in terms of their quality and usefulness for decision making. The Checklist considers the study population, intervention/treatment, comparator(s), outcome(s), covariates and analysis.

EXPLANATION

The Checklist was developed from a review of the literature with guidance from recognized experts in this field. The GRACE Initiative has been spearheaded by Quintiles Outcome in collaboration with the National Pharmaceutical Council. GRACE contributors represent perspectives from academic, government and private sectors in the US, Europe, Asia and Africa. A listing of contributors and collaborators can be found at www.graceprinciples.org.

VALUE AND USE

As patient registries are prospective observational cohort studies, the GRACE Checklist should be applied to any patient registry which seeks to make assessments of comparative effectiveness.

ISSUES

Approaches to scoring are currently under consideration.

BIBLIOGRAPHY

Dreyer NA, Schneeweiss S, McNeil BJ, et al. GRACE principles: recognizing high-quality observational studies of comparative effectiveness. *Am J Manag Care*. 2010;16:467-471.

Dreyer NA. Making observational studies count: shaping the future of comparative effectiveness research. *Epidemiology*. 2011;22:295-297.

Dreyer NA, Tunis SR, Berger M, et al. Why observational studies should be among the tools used in comparative effectiveness research. *Health Affairs*. 2010;29:1818-1825.

GRACE. Good Research for Comparative Effectiveness. www.graceprinciples.org. Accessed April 24, 2013.

Berger ML, Dreyer N, Anderson Fred, et al. Prospective Observational Studies to Assess Comparative Effectiveness: The ISPOR Good Research Practices Task Force Report. *Value Health*. 2012;15:217-230.

STROBE (STrengthening the Reporting of OBservational studies in Epidemiology)

BRIEF DEFINITION

The main purpose of STROBE is to provide recommendations to improve the quality of reporting of observational studies, and to guide the planning and design of studies.

EXPLANATION

The STROBE initiative was established in 2004 by a group of methodologists, researchers and editors, including several people involved in CONSORT, who considered empirical evidence and theoretical principles relating to the reporting of observational studies. The STROBE Statement is a checklist of 22 items considered essential for good reporting of observational studies, with items specific to the 3 main study designs: cohort studies, case-control studies and cross-sectional studies (*see term:* General Study Design). The 22 items fall into the following broad categories:

- Title and abstract;
- Introduction: background/rationale, objectives;
- Methods: study design, setting, participants (cohort, case-control, and cross-sectional study), variables, data sources/measurement, bias, study size, quantitative variables, statistical methods;
- Results: participants, descriptive data, outcome data, main results, other analysis;
- Discussion: key results, limitations, interpretation, generalizability;
- Other information: funding.

VALUE AND USE

The STROBE Statement can provide assistance to authors when writing up analytical observational studies, support editors and reviewers when considering such articles for publication, and can help readers critically appraise published articles.

ISSUES

STROBE does not provide detailed information on safety evaluations. In addition, the checklist is not intended to be used as a quality scoring instrument for studies; it is limited to evaluating the quality of study reporting.

BIBLIOGRAPHY

STROBE Statement. Strengthening the reporting of observational studies in epidemiology. http://www.strobe-statement.org/. Accessed April 24, 2013.

von Elm E, Altman DG, Egger M, et al. The Strengthening the Reporting of Observational Studies in Epidemiology (STROBE) statement: guidelines for reporting observational studies. *J Clin Epidemiol*. 2008;61:344-349.

Malta M, Cardoso LO, Bastos FI, et al. Guidelines on reporting observational studies. *Rev Saude Publica*. 2010;44:559-565.

Berger ML, Dreyer N, Anderson Fred, et al. Prospective Observational Studies to Assess Comparative Effectiveness: The ISPOR Good Research Practices Task Force Report. *Value Health*. 2012;15:217-230.

SECTION III

Analysis and Reporting of Patient Registry Data

Analysis

Analysis Plan

BRIEF DEFINITION

A detailed plan, developed prior to beginning data analysis, which describes the variables, data handling, and statistical techniques used to produce results.

EXPLANATION

An analysis plan describes the analytical procedures and statistical techniques that will be used to evaluate the primary and, if applicable, secondary objectives specified in the study protocol or plan. It is also called the SAP.

VALUE AND USE

Accurate and specific reporting of the analysis plan has a positive impact on the utility and applicability of registry data. In economic evaluations of registry studies, clear descriptions of the analysis plan are helpful in translating clinical results to economic outcomes. More critically, *a priori* specification of the primary end point, and the patient and site covariates to be adjusted for, is necessary to reduce bias.

ISSUES

A registry may require a primary master SAP, as well as subsequent, supplemental SAPs. Supplemental SAPs might be triggered by new research questions emerging after the initial master SAP was developed, or because the registry evolved over time. Both master SAP and supplemental SAPs should be described in resulting publications.

BIBLIOGRAPHY

Chapter 13. Analysis and interpretation of registry data to evaluate outcomes. In: Gliklich RE, Dreyer NA, eds. *Registries for Evaluating Patient Outcomes: A User's Guide*. 2nd ed. (Prepared by Outcome DEcIDE Center [Outcome Sciences, Inc. d/b/a Outcome] under contract no. HHSA290200500351 T03.) AHRQ Publication No. 10-EHC049. Rockville, MD: Agency for Healthcare Research and Quality; 2010:285-304.

Statistical Inference and Hypothesis Testing

BRIEF DEFINITION

Statistical inference relates to the analytic techniques which evaluate whether a statistic or relationship observed in a study dataset will also be found in the population from which that dataset was taken.

EXPLANATION

In this section we are referring to 95% confidence intervals (CIs) and p-values. It is beyond the scope of this book to explain the sampling distribution theory which underlies the logic of these tools. However, this theory requires that the dataset analyzed contains persons (or other observations) which are representative of the population, and that the data collection itself does not distort population characteristics. Typically such data would be collected using random sampling, potentially with a stratification technique.

VALUE AND USE

It is important to consider statistical inference and hypothesis testing in the development of the analytic plan as these questions will guide the development of the plan (*see term:* Analysis Plan).

ISSUES

While statistical inference and hypothesis testing are critical elements to discerning associations and a potential step in the causal pathway, one cannot discount that observational studies are also developed to shed light on the development of hypotheses (*see term:* General Study Design).

BIBLIOGRAPHY

Kirkwood BR, Sterne JAC. *Essential Medical Statistics*. 2nd ed. Blackwell Publishing; 2003.

Plans-Rubio P, Payakachat N. Statistical methods for randomized controlled trials: Hypothesis testing. In: Esposito D, ed. *Reliability and Validity of Data Sources for Outcomes Research & Disease and Health Management Programs*. Lawrenceville, NJ: ISPOR; 2013:362-366.

Confidence Intervals

BRIEF DEFINITION

CIs are parameters around the point estimate reflecting the variation in the estimate by some percentage, typically 95%.

EXPLANATION

CIs are probably easier to understand than hypothesis tests despite being more information rich. The 95% CI can be calculated for almost any estimate from a dataset, whether the estimate be a mean, a mean between-group difference, the slope of a line linking 2 measurements (eg, bodyweight and age), or for a proportion. To calculate the 95% CI around a mean, the following formula is applied:

- Lower bound: mean – (1.96 · standard error of mean)
- Upper bound: mean + (1.96 · standard error of mean)

The standard error of the mean is calculated as $\frac{sd}{\sqrt{n}}$. The 1.96 scaling factor relates to an assumption derived from sampling distribution theory.

Standard errors and CIs differ from measures of spread such as the standard deviation or interquartile range. Rather than representing the spread of *observed* values in the data, confidence intervals use information about the observed spread, and the sample size, to estimate a *range of values* in which the true population average may lie. The default is to apply a scaling factor, in this case 1.96, which causes this range to have a 95% probability of including the true population value.

Standard errors and CIs are also calculable for other statistics, such as regression coefficients and odds ratios. While such calculations tend to be more complicated than the example above, the same principle applies and the derived confidence intervals serve the same purpose in terms of inference. The width of the CI has special significance if it is evaluated against some threshold. For example, the CI for a change in bodyweight following diet pill therapy is perfectly capable of including the possibility that the pill causes weight loss as well as weight gain; in this case the threshold value for mean weight change would be zero (0) kg.

VALUE AND USE

CIs provide a necessary measure of the variance and distribution of the estimate beyond the point estimate.

ISSUES

As the equation above demonstrates, the 95% CI is sensitive to the spread observed in the analyzed dataset, as well as the sample size. In general, larger samples will produce narrower CIs, as will samples whose measurements exhibit less spread, ie, smaller standard deviations (*see term:* Summary Statistics for Quantitative Variables).

BIBLIOGRAPHY

Kirkwood BR, Sterne JAC. *Essential Medical Statistics*. 2nd ed. Blackwell Publishing; 2003.

Plans-Rubio P, Payakachat N. Statistical methods for randomized controlled trials: Hypothesis testing. In: Esposito D, ed. *Reliability and Validity of Data Sources for Outcomes Research & Disease and Health Management Programs*. Lawrenceville, NJ: ISPOR; 2013:362-366.

Hypothesis Testing and P-values

BRIEF DEFINITION

Hypothesis testing is an approach by which an investigator seeks to test a hypothesis and either rejects or confirms the null hypothesis based on study data. P-values are values set by the investigator to confirm that the findings of the test do not occur merely by chance. The social science and biological literatures varies this level between .20 and .001, whereas the fields of clinical medicine, epidemiology and health economics typically use the 0.05 level as the threshold defining significance; values below this threshold indicate the estimate is not associated with chance and those above suggest that it is potentially associated with chance.

EXPLANATION

In the context of CIs discussed above, hypothesis tests use identical principles and very similar calculations to evaluate a specific research question, and test the observed data against a predefined null hypothesis. The null hypothesis typically reflects a situation of no effect, eg, no association of 2 variables, no difference in the mean of 2 groups, a mean which is unremarkable, or zero change in mean bodyweight after diet pill therapy.

Hypothesis testing revolves around the calculation of a probability, a p-value. This p-value reflects the probability that the observed estimate (eg, mean, mean difference, regression coefficient or odds ratio) could have arisen in a population in which the null hypothesis is true. Typically we would accept our result as statistically significant (*see term:* Summary Statistics for Quantitative Variables) if the p value is <0.05. This corresponds to our being "95% confident" that the observed estimate did not arise by chance and that the true situation in the population is not defined by the null hypothesis.

VALUE AND USE

The 2 inferential techniques described are essential tools in assessing the statistical robustness of findings from a dataset. Specifically they allow the researcher to determine: a) whether or not the results observed could have occurred due to chance alone rather than because of some genuine effect in the population and; b) the extent to which statistical uncertainty around the results in the dataset affects our understanding of the magnitude of a likely true effect present in the population.

ISSUES

P-values and CIs provide specific information about an effect observed in a dataset—namely, how transferable the effect is to a wider population, and how much of a role chance might be playing in the results seen. Statistical inference, in particular p-values, is commonly misused as a proxy for importance, indeed some reports focus only on the results which are statistically significant and pay little attention to the effect size itself or the width of confidence intervals. This approach is ill-advised, since 1 in 20 hypothesis tests is likely to turn up statistically significant results by chance alone, unless some arithmetic correction is applied.

When interpreting results of inference statistics, especially p-values, it must be borne in mind that statistical significance (*see term:* Summary Statistics for Quantitative Variables), attained when p is less than 0.05, reflects only that the effect observed did not arise by chance alone. It does not rule out that chance contributed partly to the observed effect. For a better understanding of how chance (that is, error, uncertainty, and sample size limitations) affect the estimated effect—consider the 95% CIs.

BIBLIOGRAPHY

Kirkwood BR, Sterne JAC. *Essential Medical Statistics.* 2nd ed. Blackwell Publishing; 2003.

Plans-Rubio P, Payakachat N. Statistical methods for randomized controlled trials: Hypothesis testing. In: Esposito D, ed. *Reliability and Validity of Data Sources for Outcomes Research & Disease and Health Management Programs.* Lawrenceville, NJ: ISPOR; 2013:362-366.

Statistical Significance Under Large Sample Sizes

BRIEF DEFINITION

Statistical significance is the quantitative degree measured by the p-value, to which a difference is likely to be obtained by chance, assuming the null hypothesis is true.

EXPLANATION

In some cases a registry is not purposefully powered to test a hypothesis and the sample size is much larger than the minimum required to test various hypotheses using the data. If a study is based on a very large sample size, relationships found to be statistically significant may not have much practical importance (clinical relevance/significance [*see term:* Hypothesis Testing and P-values]).

VALUE AND USE

Rejection of a null hypothesis by a statistical test can be meaningless if the sample size is extremely large. Therefore it may be necessary to look at measures of effect size, which take into consideration both the size of the difference and the variability of sample values, before reaching conclusions about the importance of experimental effects. Effect size can be calculated by taking the difference between the 2 groups (mean of the treatment group *minus* the mean of the control group) and dividing it by the standard deviation of 1 of the groups.

ISSUES

Unfortunately, a common misunderstanding is that a statistically significant result is always of clinical significance, or demonstrates a large effect in the population.

Given a too large sample, extremely small and nonnotable differences can be found to be statistically significant, but this says nothing about the practical significance of a difference. Therefore, attention must be paid to the minimum clinically important difference (MCID) to more fully interpret results from patient registries with large sample sizes.

BIBLIOGRAPHY

Cohen J. *Statistical Power Analysis for the Behavioral Sciences*. 2nd ed. Hillsdale, NJ: Lawrence Erlbaum Associates; 1988.

Zimmerman DW. Anomalous statistical significance associated with large N's, zero effect size, and "almost independent" observations. http://mypage.direct.ca/z/zimmerma/zeroeffectsize.html. Accessed April 24, 2013.

Multiplicity Adjustments

BRIEF DEFINITION

Multiplicity adjustments are the process of adjusting for multiple statistical tests to correct for occurrence of false positives (ie, type 1 error) that could emerge from investigators looking at many additional end points and treatment group comparisons. These adjustments offer protection against conclusions that are driven by excessive data mining that occurs when statistical tests are used repeatedly. The adjustment process effectively raises the standard of proof needed when examining a wide range of hypotheses simultaneously. Adjustment for multiple comparisons may be accomplished in many different ways. The simplest and most intuitive approach is the Bonferroni method. Other methods to adjust for multiple comparisons include the Holm, Hochberg, hierarchical testing, and bootstrap methods. See below for the explanation of each of these methods. The main purpose of using any of these methods is to rule out chance as a possible explanation for observed findings in a clinical trial or observational study.

EXPLANATION

Accurate data analysis and interpretation of findings are important to every policy maker who needs statistical data to inform decision making. In recent times, computing technologies used in analyzing data are relatively inexpensive and readily available to researchers. As a result, investigators question and analyze data from every possible dimension. The result of such extensive data analysis is the increased chance of reporting inaccurate findings from medical interventions in clinical trials or observational studies. Multiplicity adjustments are used to correct for such extensive data mining and to rule out chance as an explanation of significant findings. The degree and also the necessity of adjusting for multiplicity in clinical trials and observational studies has been an issue for a long time, with differing opinion among researchers. It has been proven in most research studies that comparing data multiple times at a significance level of 0.05 often increases the chance of committing at least a single type 1 error, otherwise known as family wise error (FWE) rate.

There are different methods of correcting for multiple testing procedures in clinical trials or observational studies. Each of these methods use slightly different algorithms in adjusting for multiple end points, multiple treatments, or multiple looks at the data. For instance, the Bonferroni method, the simplest and most intuitive approach, requires that the p-value for each comparison be less than or equal to 0.05 divided by the total number of study comparisons. This approach guarantees that the probability of at least one type I error (FWE) is less than 0.05. The Bonferroni method is the most commonly used adjustment, serves as the benchmark, and is more conservative. On the other hand, the Hochberg false discovery rate (FDR) method is the least stringent among other methods and has the propensity to produce false positive outcomes. The Holm correction method is very similar to the Bonferroni method with the exception that it is less conservative. It is known as the Bonferroni step-down. The FWE rates in both the Bonferroni and Holm methods are similar. These methods are considered to be single-step procedures. In the Holm method, the p-value of each comparison is ranked from the smallest to the largest. The Westfall and Young Permutation (Hierarchical Testing) is another multiple correction method that uses a step-wise approach. This method is considered to be more powerful than the single-step approach. The method follows a step-down procedure similar to the Holm method. The bootstrap method creates pseudodatasets by sampling observations with replacement from a pool of interventions. The permutation method also creates a pseudodataset by dividing the data into artificial treatment and control groups. This process is repeated multiple times in both the bootstrap (*see term:* Bootstrap) and permutations methods. The bootstrap method explicitly incorporates all sources of correlation, including multiple contrasts and multivariate structure. The adjusted p-values incorporate all correlations and distributional characteristics. Because of these characteristics, resampling methods tend to be less conservative than the other methods.

VALUE AND USE

Although multiplicity adjustments are controversial, in recent years they have gained acceptance in various scientific fields. It is considered important in pharmaceutical safety determinations involving multiple end points and with multiple cohorts/treatment arms in clinical trials. For instance, the postmenopausal estrogen/progestin intervention study is usually considered a good example of a conservative trial in which one of the adjustment methods (Bonferroni) was widely used to adjust for multiplicity arising from both multiple end points and multiple study treatments. These methods are used to help in the collective evaluation of several independent studies having similar designs. This approach helps find a probable solution which achieves optimal power for a certain error in decision and a specified set of alternatives. For example, the regulatory guidelines on use of PROs to support medical product labeling claims recommend adjusting for multiple comparisons in PRO. The SAS® procedure called PROC MULTTEST was developed to address multiplicity concerns in clinical trials and other observational studies and is used to perform multiplicity adjustment. The PROC MULTTEST calculates adjusted p-values for any of the multiplicity adjustment methods supplied by the user.

Multiplicity adjustments are also important in epidemiology, health services research, and other sophisticated areas of data analysis, as they offer protection against conclusions that are driven by excessive data mining. Some of the main advantages of adopting the multiplicity-adjustment approach are as follows:

- Allows data analysts to calculate the maximum amount of α error possible with any overall hypothesis.
- The approach is flexible because it allows data analysts to choose a cutoff point for p value.
- Helps in maintaining internal consistency and also reduces errors in decision making.
- Provides scope for a certain degree of variability.
- Can be used in analyzing correlated data.

ISSUES

The effects of multiple data manipulation and tests are real and important. If not properly handled, the multiplicity problem often results in increasing numbers of false positives and thus creates a false illusion of the effectiveness of an intervention. It has been suggested that if not properly controlled, multiplicity can potentially cause 3 kinds of problems: 1) declaring a treatment to be statistically significant when it's truly not, 2) declaring effects of an intervention in the wrong direction, and, 3) inflating the true effect of an intervention. Among these 3 issues, the major concern is the inflation of scientific findings. These concerns notwithstanding, there is currently a trend to discount the multiplicity problem and its effects. Some agree that there is no need to adjust for multiple comparisons. Without adjustment, the methods protect against the global null hypothesis that no treatment has any effect and no subgroup benefits from treatment. On the other hand, some investigators believe that it is safer to adjust than to report erroneous statistical significant results, particularly in clinical trials.

Although several studies have elaborated on types of adjustment procedures available, there have been very few studies that have described specific conditions that demand the use of multiplicity adjustment as a control measure. There have been numerous arguments floating around as to where the line of separation for the use and nonuse of multiplicity adjustment needs to be drawn. For example, some statisticians have argued that "It seems ironic that when many investigators publish their separate findings in the medical literature, per-comparison error rates are routinely accepted. However, when one investigator takes on the entire job, the same approach may no longer be deemed valid." On the other hand are conservative statisticians who use the multiplicity adjustment for almost everything.

Because there are many issues that either separately or in combination may make a coherent case for or against the multiplicity adjustment, most statisticians and other investigators recommend the following:

- Reduce the number of comparisons as a solution to multiplicity.
- Consider the degree of controversy when multiplicity adjustment is being contemplated.
- Even though definitive conclusions regarding the necessity for multiplicity adjustment may not be clear in each case, the issues concerning the relevance of the adjustment for each scenario are brought into focus and discussed.
- Consider who stands to benefit from the multiplicity, and the nature of the study/alternative hypothesis. For example, does a single entity, such as a manufacturer, gain from making multiple comparisons? If so, they are open to the criticism that multiplicity was deliberately introduced to give more opportunities to declare a treatment benefit which otherwise may not be true. In this case, it gives the appearance that multiplicity was used to increase the chance of stopping the trial and declaring benefit.
- Finally, statisticians encourage the presentation of interval estimation (eg, relative risks with CIs (*see term:* Confidence Interval) for effects rather than just hypothesis testing (*see term:* Hypothesis Testing and p values) (eg, p value).

In the midst of all the controversy surrounding the use of multiplicity adjustments, it should be noted that the one reason behind the application of these methods is to rule out chance as the cause of significant findings in either a clinical trial or observational studies.

BIBLIOGRAPHY

Proschan MA, Waclawiw MA. Practical guidelines for multiplicity adjustment in clinical trials. *Control Clin Trials.* 2000;21:527-539.

Leon AC, Heo M, Teres JJ, Morikawa T. Statistical power of multiplicity adjustment strategies for correlated binary endpoints. *Statist Med.* 2007;26:1712-1723.

Schulz KF, Grimes DA. Multiplicity in randomised trials I: endpoints and treatments. *Lancet.* 2005;365:1591-1595.

Westfall P, Bretz F. Multiplicity in clinical trials. In: Chow SC, ed. *Encyclopedia of Biopharmaceutical Statistics.* 2nd ed. New York, NY: Marcel Dekker; 2003:666-673.

Patrick DL, Burke LB, Powers JH, et al. Patient-reported outcomes to support medical product labeling claims: FDA perspective. *Value Health.* 2007;10:S125-S137.

Miller VT, LaRosa J, Barnabei V, et al. Effects of estrogen or estrogen/progestin regimens on heart disease risk factors in postmenopausal women: the Postmenopausal Estrogen/Progestin Interventions (PEPI) trial. *JAMA.*1995;273:199-208.

Benjamini Y, Hochberg Y. Controlling the false discovery rate: a practical and powerful approach to multiple testing. *J R Statist Soc B.* 1995;57:289-300.

Holm S. A simple sequentially rejective multiple test procedure. *Scand J Statist.* 1979;6:65-70.

Hommel G. A stagewise rejective multiple test procedure based on a modified Bonferroni test. *Biometrika*. 1988;75:383-386.
Hochberg Y. A sharper Bonferroni procedure for multiple tests of significance. *Biometrika*. 1998;75:800-803.
Tukey JW. Some thoughts on clinical trials, especially problems of multiplicity. *Science*. 1977;198:679-684.
Perneger TV. What's wrong with Bonferroni adjustments. *BMJ*. 1998;316:1236-1238.

Available Variables for Analyses

BRIEF DEFINITION

Variables for analyses refer to the parameters employed in statistical analysis and are defined by the study objectives.

EXPLANATION

Variables for analyses can be classified into the following types:

» *Quantitative Variables*

Any variable that is naturally measured as a number for which meaningful arithmetic operations can be employed is a quantitative variable. Quantitative variables are usually summarized by some estimate of an average or typical value, as well as by overviews of the spread of observations, eg, variance around this average (*see term:* Summary Statistics for Quantitative Variables). Quantitative variables can be further classified as continuous and count variables.

» *Continuous*

A quantitative variable that takes any value in a certain interval is a continuous variable. Patient's age, body mass index, height, weight, waist-to-hip ratio, etc., could be examples of continuous clinical variables used in registries. Likewise, hospital and surgeon volume per year could be one of the provider performance-related variables used in registries. A continuous variable can be described in terms of median, mean and standard deviation (*see term:* Summary Statistics for Quantitative Variables).

» *Count*

Any variable that consists of only a countable number of distinct values is a count/discrete variable. For example, number of comorbidities.

» *Categorical Variables*

Any variable that is not quantitative in nature can be called a categorical variable. A categorical variable with 2 modalities is known as a dichotomous variable. A categorical variable can be obtained from transforming any quantitative variable into class intervals. Categorical variables can be further classified as nominal/qualitative and ordinal.

» *Nominal/Qualitative/Dichotomous*

A nominal variable is purely a name variable where no ordering relationship exists between the values of the variable. Nominal variables are also referred to as qualitative variables (*see term:* Summary Statistics for Qualitative Variables). For example, gender (binary), race/ethnicity, marital status, and geographical region are examples of nominal, qualitative variables. Nominal or qualitative variables can be described in many dichotomous categories, such as binary (yes/no), or multinomial (married, divorced, widowed, single, etc.).

» *Ordinal*

An ordinal variable is a type of categorical variable for which the levels of the variable can be naturally rank ordered. Examples of ordinal variables include levels of education, ratings and rankings of levels of treatment satisfaction, physical and mental component scales of the 36-Item Short Form Health Survey (SF-36), the general well-being scale, etc.

Categorical variables can be described with frequency tables and cross-tabulations which consist of counting the number of individuals per modality or a combination of modalities.

Additionally, depending upon the study objective, the above-mentioned variables can be used as outcome variable(s) of interest, independent variable(s), and covariates (*see term:* Confounders/Covariates) for the purpose of analysis.

» *Outcome(s) of Interest*

Outcome is a response variable one would be interested in predicting. An outcome variable is also known as a dependent variable (*see term:* Analysis Techniques). Common outcomes of interest include, in-hospital mortality (a dichotomous variable; 0= died, 1=survived), health care expenditures (continuous variable), number of physician visits (count variable), etc. The outcome variable is mathematically denoted by Y. In registries, intermediate outcomes or biomarkers such as hemoglobin A1C levels in diabetes or viral load/sustained virological response in chronic hepatitis C, both reflective of final long-term outcomes, could also be used.

» *Independent Variables*

An independent variable is one that explains the response/outcome variable in a study. An independent variable is also known as an explanatory variable or predictor or exposure variable (in an epidemiologic study). For example, surgeon volume (ie, number of procedures performed per year) could be categorized into a 3-level ordinal variable: low, medium, and high volume and used to predict an outcome of interest.

» *Confounders/Covariates*

Confounders or covariates are variables that might impact the outcome variable, while distorting the true relationship/association between the independent variable(s) and the outcome variable(s). For example, age (can be used as continuous, or categorical if grouped) and gender (dichotomous variable 0= female, 1= male) are common covariates in analyses.

The functional relationship between independent and dependent variables can be denoted as:

$Y= f(X)$

where Y is the dependent variable and X the independent variable.

In general, the dependent variable, independent variable, and covariates can be expressed in a multiple regression equation format as:

$Y= \beta_0 + \beta_1 X_1 + \beta_{(2\text{-}k)} X(2\text{-}k) + \varepsilon.$

where Y is the dependent variable,

X, and $X_{(2\text{-}k)}$ are independent variables;

k is the number of independent variables;

β_0 is the intercept;

β_1 and $\beta_{(2\text{-}k)}$ are parameters that measure the change in expected value of Y, E(Y), as the respective X, and $X_{(2\text{-}k)}$ increases by 1 with all the other independent variables held fixed; and,

ε is the error term in the model.

Statistically, the relationship between the dependent and the independent variable can be described using a scatter plot.

Typically in registries, data are collected on patient characteristics that are time invariant (demographics such as gender and race) and time variant such as baseline patient characteristics (clinical measurements, patient reported outcomes), follow-up clinical and patient-reported data not necessarily collected at predefined time intervals, and health care utilization (inpatient visits, emergency room visits, laboratory tests, prescription drug fills, and physician visits (*see term:* Data: Sources, Elements, Capture and Quality Assurance)). For example, the Severe Chronic Neutropenia International Registry (SCNIR), established in 1994, contains retrospectively transferred clinical trial data from 1987 to 1994 and prospectively collected data for newly diagnosed SCN patients from 1994 onward. Some of the variables collected and analyzed periodically (usually annually) include patient demographics (age, sex, race/ethnicity, city, state, and country), clinical characteristics (type and frequency of infectious episodes, type and frequency of noninfectious clinical events, physical assessments), treatment variables (applied therapies, side-effects of treatment, treatment safety, nonresponsiveness), secondary events (incidence of leukemia, bone marrow transplant) and the final outcome of death.

VALUE AND USE

The Analysis Techniques section covers the main ways in which single variables may be summarized and used in analysis of registry data (*see term:* Analysis Techniques).

ISSUES

Sometimes there are fewer variables available in registries compared to clinical trials. Also, because patient registries are designed to capture data in the real world with minimal research interference, the degree of measurement precision and standardization of measures is often lower than in clinical trials. For example, a clinical trial collecting data on patient body weight may mandate that all weight scales at investigator sites be calibrated, or even that identical/similar scales be used across the trial. Patient registries generally make no such demand on the research sites.

BIBLIOGRAPHY

Woolson RF. *Statistical Methods for the Analysis of Biomedical Data*. New York, NY: Wiley Series; 1987.

Dale DC, Bolyard AA, Schwinzer BG, et al. The Severe Chronic Neutropenia International Registry: 10-year follow-up report. *Support Cancer Ther.* 2006;3:220-231.

Munro BH. *Statistical Methods for Health Care Research*. 4th ed. Philadelphia, PA: Lippincott Williams & Wilkins; 2000.

Hay J. Statistical approaches and methods. In: Esposito D, ed. *Reliability and Validity of Data Sources for Outcomes Research & Disease and Health Management Programs*. Lawrenceville, NJ: ISPOR; 2013:335-433.

Missing Observations

BRIEF DEFINITION

Missing observations are a major challenge to the success and interpretation of research results. Missing observations are essentially a lack of response. This can happen at any stage of clinical or observational research and to any extent, from a participant dropping out of the study completely (due to AEs/lost to follow up, etc.) to being unable to answer, or refusing to answer, certain questions on PROs. Missing observation can also occur when respondents cannot understand/interpret the response (ie, a "don't know" response, or unreadable or ambiguous answers (eg, 2 responses circled [*see term:* Data Capture/Collection]).

EXPLANATION

With small datasets, even small amounts of missing observations can cause problems in interpretation and analysis. When the amount of missing data becomes large, study results can become inconclusive. The important question to ask with missing observations is "Does an underlying true value exist?" Missing observations (missing data) potentially introduce bias and interfere with the ability to compare effects across clinical trial arms or, in the case of patient registries, patient cohorts. Because only a subset of the initial population contributes data, there is a loss of statistical power. In addition, the patient cohorts with data may no longer be systematically comparable to those at baseline due to data missing in a nonrandom fashion. Missing data (and the dropout mechanism) should be interpreted as a potential outcome in its own right as it can be considered a surrogate for patient preference or acceptability with therapy, and is potentially nonpredictive of where the study participant would be in the future (where no observations are taken or available [*see term:* Loss to Follow-up]).

Missing observations fall into 3 categories:

» ***Missing Completely at Random (MCAR)***

MCAR occurs when the likelihood of an observation being missing is unrelated to the value of this observation or to the value of other variables, $Pr\{M|Y_O,Y_M, X\} = Pr\{M|X\}$, where M=missing; Y_O=value of observed record of interest; YM=true value of missing/unobserved record of interest, X=value of other records.

» ***Missing at Random (MAR)***

MAR occurs when the likelihood of an observation being missing does not depend on the value of the missing observation after controlling for another variable(s), $Pr\{M|Y_O,Y_M, X\} = Pr\{M|Y_O,X\}$

» ***Missing Not at Random (MNAR)***

MNAR occurs when the likelihood of an observation being missing depends on the value of the dropped-out observation. $Pr\{M|Y_M\}$

VALUE AND USE

The inclusion of patient-completed questionnaires in clinical and observational research adds another level of complexity to missing data, as participants may choose not to complete, or be unable to complete, a questionnaire or selected questionnaire items. An example item would be family income if the response were to reveal either a particularly low- or high-income amount. Such missing data is a possible indication of unacceptable patient burden or inappropriate items or response options.

ISSUES

If missing observations are associated with treatment effects that cannot be predicted from measurements on patients with complete data, then the treatment effect (*see term:* Treatment Effects Models and Instrumental Variables) obtained based on missing imputations will be biased.

BIBLIOGRAPHY

Rubin DB. Inference and missing data. *Biometrika*. 1976;63:581-592.

Little RJA, Rubin DB. *Statistical Analysis with Missing Data*. New York, NY: John Wiley; 1987.

Allison PD. Multiple imputation for missing data: a cautionary tale. *Social Methods Res*. 2000;28:301-309.

Allison PD. *Missing Data*. Thousand Oaks, CA: Sage; 2002.

Luo R. Statistical methods for randomized controlled trials: missing data in outcomes research studies. In: Esposito D, ed. *Reliability and Validity of Data Sources for Outcomes Research & Disease and Health Management Programs*. Lawrenceville, NJ: ISPOR; 2013:393-397.

Strategies for Handling Missing Observations

BRIEF DEFINITION

Multiple strategies exist for the treatment of missing data. The appropriate strategy for the imputation of missing observations may depend on the type of missing observation as introduced and defined in the previous section.

A variety of statistical strategies have been proposed in the literature to deal with missing observations due to patient withdrawal from assigned treatment exposure prior to planned completion of the trial. These enable every patient randomized to contribute some observation to the analysis and are summarized below. Imputation is a common strategy for handling missing data utilizing either average value substitution with unconditional or conditional means, or hot-deck (ie, missing value is imputed from a randomly selected similar record within the same dataset) or cold-deck (ie, missing value is imputed from a similar record from another, different dataset) imputations, or for data on multiple time points, using last observation carried forward, or more recently, multiple imputations. Importantly, no single method is generally accepted or preferred. Imputation of missing data is done on a per-patient basis and tries to predict missing observations using data from patients for whom all data have been collected. This involves assumptions about what caused data and observations to be missing, which usually cannot be verified from the data. If missing observations are associated with treatment effects in ways that cannot be predicted from measurements on subjects with complete data, analyses using imputation procedures, and conclusions about treatment impact, will be biased. The FDA therefore encourages the collection of data on each patient at the time of withdrawal to determine the reason for withdrawal. When available, this information can be taken into account in the analysis.

EXPLANATION

Potential strategies to address each of the 3 types of missing data are as follows:

» *Strategies when Data is MCAR*

Analysis of complete cases. With this approach, no imputation is performed and the analysis is conducted solely on those records with complete cases. The advantage to this approach is that it is simple to describe and easy to implement; the disadvantage is that it is inefficient, as there is a loss of information contained in those incomplete cases.

Single imputation. In this approach, the missing observation is imputed. The advantage to this approach is that it is relatively simple to implement; the disadvantage is that the imputation itself may be based on unrealistic assumptions and/or generate biased estimates. The most common single imputation method is Last Observation Carried Forward (LOCF). LOCF is a method of imputing missing observations by carrying the previous observed value forward. For example, if weight was missing at week 4, the LOCF value for weight at week 4 is the weight at week 3, provided weight was measured and nonmissing at week 3. However, LOCF can be problematic for the following reasons: (1) If the objective of the trial or study is to detect a treatment effect after a certain duration of treatment (eg, at 4 weeks), then a comparison that includes only measurements on patients at earlier times or visits is not addressing the original trial or study objective. The average of patient responses, many of which are at different times or visits, may be uninterpretable; (2) LOCF makes an implicit assumption that the patient would sustain the same response seen at an early study visit for the entire duration of the trial or study. This assumption is untestable and potentially unrealistic.

Generalized Estimating Equations (GEE). For models fitted with GEEs, observations with missing values within a cluster are not used, and all available pairs are used in estimating the working correlation matrix. GEE is used to fit the parameters of a generalized linear model where unknown correlation is present (*see term:* Generalized Estimating Equations). The GEE allows for correlation without explicitly defining a model for the origin of the dependency, hence it is most suitable when the random effects and their variances are not of direct interest. SAS procedures for GEE include SAS® PROC GENMOD (with REPEATED= statement). PROC GENMOD ignores any observation with a missing value for any variable involved in the model. GEE is often used for longitudinal data and generally requires MCAR or covariate-dependent dropout in order to yield consistent estimates.

» *Strategies when Data is MAR*

Multiple imputations. In this method a series of values for each missing observation are generated using an estimated distribution (Rubin 1987). This method involves simulating possible values of the missing data and constructing multiple datasets. Then, a model is estimated using each new dataset and the means of parameters across the samples are computed. Standard errors can be obtained via a combination of the between-model variance and the within-model standard errors. Although this approach adjusts for the downward bias that some of the previous approaches produce, its key drawbacks are that it assumes the data are MAR, and it is fairly difficult to implement. Procedures in SAS include SAS® PROC MI and PROC MIANALYZE.

Mixed models. Mixed models encompass models with multiple sources of variation such as are found in hierarchical experimental designs, models where treatments may alter the variability of the responses as well as the mean of the responses, and models for repeated measures trials with complicated variance structures. In this approach, no attempt is made to impute or estimate missing values. Procedures in SAS include SAS® PROC MIXED or PROC NLMIXED.

» *Strategies when Data is MNAR*

This strategy involves statistical treatments that are based on the distributions of {YO,YM} and M, where M=missing; YO=value of observed record of interest; YM=true value of missing/unobserved record of interest.

Pattern-mixture models. These models stratify the data according to time to dropout and formulate a model for each stratum. Pattern-mixture models are frequently used for longitudinal data analysis with dropouts because they do not require explicit specification of the dropout mechanism.

Selection models. Selection models model p(Y,Observed) = p(Observed | Y) p(Y). The classic 2-step method for which Heckman won the Nobel Prize involves a) estimating a selection equation; b) constructing a new variable—a hazard for sample inclusion—that is a function of predicted scores from this model, c) including this new variable in the structural model of interest.

VALUE AND USE

The statistical strategies described above are used to impute missing observations due to patient withdrawal from assigned treatment prior to completion of a clinical trial or prospective observational study. The specific strategy applied depends on the type of missing data.

ISSUES

There is no single general imputation method that is preferred. Regardless of the imputation technique, imputed values are estimates of the unknown true values. Thus, any analysis that ignores the uncertainty of predicted missing data will lead to smaller standard errors, artificially smaller p-values, and higher type I error rates (*see term:* Multiplicity Adjustments).

BIBLIOGRAPHY

Rubin DB. Inference and missing data. *Biometrika*. 1976;63:581-592.

Little RJA, Rubin DB. *Statistical Analysis with Missing Data*. New York, NY: John Wiley; 1987.

Allison PD. Multiple imputation for missing data: a cautionary tale. *Social Methods Res*. 2000;28: 301-309.

Allison PD. *Missing Data*. Thousand Oaks, CA: Sage; 2002.

Guo W, Ratcliffe SJ, Ten Have TT. A random pattern-mixture model for longitudinal data with dropouts. *J Amer Statistical Assoc*. 2004;99:929-937.

Luo R. Statistical methods for randomized controlled trials: missing data in outcomes research studies. In: Esposito D, ed. *Reliability and Validity of Data Sources for Outcomes Research & Disease and Health Management Programs*. Lawrenceville, NJ: ISPOR; 2013:393-397.

Timing of Analyses

Interim Analysis

BRIEF DEFINITION

An interim analysis refers to an analysis taking place at a time point when not all of the data have been collected. This time point can be determined *a priori* at the development of the analysis plan (*see term:* Analysis Plan) or can be *ad hoc* based on some new information or activity that raises concern or questions about the data.

EXPLANATION

Interim analyses may be planned prior to study commencement but may also simply be checks carried out along the way to ensure the data collection is proceeding as expected or that the treatment being observed is not causing undue safety concerns.

VALUE AND USE

The interim analysis provides significant value to the investigators because many observational studies (*see term:* General Study Design) and registries have long follow-up periods. An interim analysis allows for the dissemination of knowledge of any potential negative or beneficial effects found to be present sooner than the completion of the study.

ISSUES

An interim analysis allows for the observation of the effect, so from a statistical perspective one must account for this multiplicative effect imposed by replicating the analysis multiple times (the concept of results occurring by chance as associated with statistical theory are affected by more than one repeat of the analysis). The use of adjustment for multiplicity (more than one replicated analysis of the data) is addressed through the use of a Bonferroni's correction or another approach and should be considered in powering the study and sample size estimation (*see term:* Multiplicity Adjustments).

BIBLIOGRAPHY

Proschan M, Waclawiw M. Practical guidelines for multiplicity adjustment in clinical trials. *Control Clin Trials*. 2000;21:527-539.

Leon AC, Heo M, Teres JJ, Morikawa T. Statistical power of multiplicity adjustment strategies for correlated binary endpoints. *Stat Med*. 2007;26:1712–1723.

Schulz KF, Grimes DA. Multiplicity in randomised trials I: endpoints and treatments. *Lancet*. 2005;365:1591-1595.

Westfall PH, Bretz F. Multiplicity in clinical trials. In: Chow SC, ed. *Encyclopedia of Biopharmaceutical Statistics*. 3rd ed. New York, NY: Marcel Dekker; 2010.

Post Hoc Analyses

BRIEF DEFINITION

The research question and its method of analysis are decided after the data have been seen, typically in response to an unexpected anomaly.

EXPLANATION

Post hoc analyses are sometimes conducted when unplanned-for confounding variables (*see term:* Confounders/Covariates) or unexpected distributions of key variables necessitate the use of alternative methods. *Post hoc* analyses are also used when performing feasibility assessments around registry analyses, eg, assessing how many observations are available for use in the registry, or identifying whether variables in the registry are adequate reflections of the variables which a potential study seeks to address.

VALUE AND USE

Post hoc analyses are meaningful and useful to maximize the use of the data and further explore other hypotheses that may have arisen from the study or from the literature (*see term:* Hypothesis Testing and P-values).

ISSUES

Post hoc analysis should not be confused with multiplicity (*see term:* Multiplicity Adjustments), as the latter is testing the same hypothesis more than once versus testing new hypotheses (*see term:* Hypothesis Testing and P-values) determined after the data has been collected and analyzed according to the analysis plan (*see term:* Analysis Plan).

BIBLIOGRAPHY

Berger VW. A priori v post hoc testing. In: Everitt BS, Howell DC, eds. *Encyclopedia of Statistics in Behavioral Science*. 1st ed. Hoboken, NJ: John Wiley & Sons; 2005.

Sensitivity Analyses

BRIEF DEFINITION

Sensitivity analysis is a way of characterizing the impact of uncertainty on the findings of a study, typically by presenting multiple scenarios for estimated or unknown variables (eg, missing patient data at baseline or follow-up), model inputs, and/or subgroup analyses.

EXPLANATION

Sensitivity analysis refers to a procedure used to determine the sensitivity of the study result to alterations of a parameter. If a small parameter alteration leads to a relatively large change in the results, the results are said to be sensitive to that parameter. This procedure may be used to determine how the final study results might change when taking into account the uncertainties in some parameters. Some sensitivity analyses, such as assessments of the outcome in a subgroup of patients, might be preplanned during the registry protocol or SAP development (*see term:* Analysis Plan).

VALUE AND USE

The results of health economics and outcomes studies are subject to a degree of uncertainty, which needs to be assessed, especially in light of the fact that such studies are frequently used in decision making. Sensitivity analyses represent a relatively easy and straightforward approach to interpreting the results and assessing the robustness of the results obtained from a particular analysis. Often, because of data limitations, sensitivity analysis represents the only tool available for assessing uncertainty around a set of results.

ISSUES

Due to the growing importance of health outcome studies in health care decision making, it is important to ensure that uncertainty is dealt with in a robust manner. Because sensitivity analysis involves significant analyst discretion (as the analyst chooses which variables to vary and the amount of variation), it is critical that good research practice be followed in this area to promote valid results. Although Briggs and Sculpher (1995) have produced guidelines for presenting the results of sensitivity analyses in economic evaluations, there are few generally agreed-upon guidelines on how to conduct or interpret sensitivity analyses in different types of health outcomes or economic studies.

BIBLIOGRAPHY

Berger ML, Bingefors K, Hedblom EC, et al, eds. *Health Care Cost, Quality, and Outcomes: ISPOR Book of Terms*. Lawrenceville, NJ: ISPOR; 2003.

Chapter 13. Analysis and interpretation of registry data to evaluate outcomes. In: Gliklich RE, Dreyer NA, eds. *Registries for Evaluating Patient Outcomes: A User's Guide*. 2nd ed. (Prepared by Outcome DEcIDE Center [Outcome Sciences, Inc. d/b/a Outcome] under contract no. HHSA290200500351 T03.) AHRQ Publication No. 10-EHC049. Rockville, MD: Agency for Healthcare Research and Quality; 2010:285-304.

Briggs A, Sculpher M. Sensitivity analysis in economic evaluation: A review of published studies. *Health Econ*. 1995;4:355-371.

Analysis Techniques

Summary Statistics for Quantitative Variables

BRIEF DEFINITION

Summary statistics are used to summarize a set of numbers. Summary statistics, or descriptive statistics, describe data characteristics to include measures of central tendency, distribution, and dispersion. Summary statistics can also be referred to as univariate analysis since it is the process by which one assesses individual variable characteristics as opposed to inferential statistics which is the comparison of multiple variables for the purposes of hypothesis testing (*see terms:* Statistical Inference and Hypothesis Testing; Summary Statistics for Quantitative Variables).

EXPLANATION

Quantitative variables are usually summarized by measures intended to reflect the average or typical value (known as central tendency) as well as the distribution of values (known as the spread or dispersion). Measures of central tendency include the mean, median, and mode, while measures of spread or dispersion include variance, standard deviation and standard error of the mean and quartiles.

The arithmetic mean is computed by adding up the values of all observations and dividing by the number of observations. It is the best understood of statistical summaries. The arithmetic mean can readily be adapted to make inferences about the underlying population from which the dataset was sampled (providing this sampling was representative, appropriately randomized and stratified where appropriate). However, it is sensitive to extreme values (eg, the presence of one billionaire in a dataset may substantially inflate the mean income computed), but this effect diminishes as sample size increases. Also, the arithmetic mean is an inappropriate summary in datasets where the observed values are not distributed at least roughly in the form of a normal distribution (or bell curve) which is centered on this mean.

The geometric mean is computed by adding up the logged (either natural or base 10) values of all observations and dividing by the number of observations, then antilogging the result. It is useful for measurements which have no naturally occurring zero, those which are very strongly right-skewed, and those whose distribution of logged values looks like a bell curve.

The median is computed as the value at which 50% of the observations have values higher, and 50% of observations have values lower. This measure is insensitive to extreme values. Where the observed values closely resemble a normal distribution (or bell curve), the median should be approximately equal to the arithmetic mean.

The mode is calculated by finding the value which occurs most frequently in the observations. This is useful for datasets where it is expected that some observations will have the same value on a variable, eg, height in centimeters. There can be more than one mode if there are several clusters of the same values. The mode is useful for checking whether the data conform to a normal distribution (bell curve). Normal distributions ought to have only one mode, and this should fall around the same value as the arithmetic mean and median.

The variance is calculated to get an idea about the average distance of the values observed to the mean. The square root of the variance is called the standard deviation (*see term:* Summary Statistics for Quantitative Variables).

The standard error of the mean (SEM) is the standard deviation of the sample mean estimate of a population mean. It can also be viewed as the standard deviation of the error in the sample mean relative to the true mean, since the sample mean is an unbiased estimator. SEM is usually estimated by the sample estimate of the sample standard deviation divided by the square root of the sample size, assuming statistical independence of the values in the sample.

The 25% and 75% quartile together with the median divide the observations into four subgroups of equal size.

VALUE AND USE

Measures of central tendency are useful for finding the typical values for a studied variable. Summary statistics are also of use in learning the basic characteristics of a population of interest, as well as for comparison between populations. Furthermore, summary statistics are a logical precursor to inferential statistics (*see term:* Statistical Inference and Tests). Before examining the predicted distribution of a variable, it is useful to look at the actual distribution. For a registry these univariate statistics are of major importance as they describe the distribution of the variable observed.

ISSUES

Descriptive statistics, particularly measures of central tendency, can be misused. Choosing the wrong measure can produce skewed results. As previously mentioned, the mean is sensitive to extreme cases. The consequence of not taking this into account is an average that is potentially much higher or lower than what is truly typical for the sample or population. Simply removing the extreme cases can lessen the generalizability of results and should be done with extreme caution. Because there is the potential to skew results by choosing the wrong measure of interest, it is important to prespecify the measures that will be used for assessing primary end points (*see term:* Analysis Plan). To overcome this issue, at least mean and median plus the standard deviation should be presented in tables of results.

BIBLIOGRAPHY

Boslaugh S, Watters PA. *Statistics in a Nutshell: A Desktop Quick Reference.* Sebastopol CA: O'Reilly Media Inc.; 2008. http://ibmstudies.com.np/files/Others/OReilly.Statistics.in.a.Nutshell.A.Desktop.Quick.Reference.Aug.2008.pdf. Accessed April 25, 2013.

Hay J. Nonparametric statistical methods. In: Esposito D, ed. *Reliability and Validity of Data Sources for Outcomes Research & Disease and Health Management Programs.* Lawrenceville, NJ: ISPOR; 2013:429-433.

Summary Statistics for Qualitative Variables

BRIEF DEFINITION

Qualitative variables are typically recorded as categories in registry datasets and are summarized by way of simple tables reporting frequencies and percentages.

EXPLANATION

Frequencies describe the number of events associated with the strata while percentages represent the fraction of the units divided by the total units in the strata. Typically percentages are reported as either row or column percentages (detailed labeling is recommended in tables to ensure correct interpretation).

VALUE AND USE

Frequencies and percentages are primarily used to describe nominal data (*see term:* Nominal/Qualitative/Dichotomous). These measures are typically more often utilized than measures of central tendency and spread when describing a population or sample, or in concert with these measures of continuous data (*see term:* Available Variables for Analyses).

ISSUES

Descriptive statistics, like measures of central tendency, can be misused. Comparison of frequencies among 2 or more strata can be misleading if the total number of units within the strata are different. Percentages allow the reader to easily see the distribution of the variable between the strata. While this does not allow the reader to compare the 2 distributions, it does allow the reader to make initial estimates about the differences between strata and the potential direction of the difference, if a difference exists.

BIBLIOGRAPHY

Wooldridge JM. *Introductory Econometrics: A Modern Approach.* 2nd ed. Cincinnati, OH: South-Western College Pub; 2002.

Munro BH. *Statistical Methods for Health Care Research.* 4th ed. Philadelphia, PA: Lippincott Williams & Wilkins; 2000.

Statistical Inference and Tests

BRIEF DEFINITION

Inferential statistics is a process by which data are used to draw inferences about a population. This process utilizes 2 approaches to testing assumptions which are the Frequentist approach and the Bayesian approach. These 2 branches of statistics differ on the use of prior information and the definition of probability which in turn affects research design, analysis and interpretation.

EXPLANATION

Bayesian analysis is an approach that utilizes information from previous events to draw generalized results from an incomplete dataset without relying on numerical interpretations to substantiate those results. It does not use p-values, nor does it test hypotheses for probability levels (*see term:* Hypothesis Testing and P-values), but rather, generates a probability that the hypothesis is true or false. The Frequentist approach, alternately, is a more common methodology which relies on repeat population sampling and the incorporation of hypothesis testing, p-values, type I and II errors and confidence intervals (*see terms:* Confidence Intervals; Multiplicity Adjustments) to establish numerical probabilities of the event in question.

VALUE AND USE

Inferential statistics allow predictions and assumptions to be drawn from a dataset and applied to the hypothesis tested. Parameters, score distributions, and distribution shapes can be estimated from the dataset and used to forecast likely results. There are 2 main types of tests that can be utilized within this branch of statistics: parametric and nonparametric. Parametric tests are used for normally distributed data and make assumptions and distribution predictions on the dataset. Other commonly used parametric distributions include the t-distribution, the Gamma-distribution or the binomial distribution. Nonparametric tests are used for non-normal data distributions and do not make assumptions or distribution predictions from the dataset.

ISSUES

Parametric tests, while more sensitive to errors and therefore more likely to have a null hypotheses rejected, still maintain results that are more significant and valid in comparison to nonparametric tests due to their more generalized nature, if the distribution of the sample aligns with the assumptions of the parametric test used (eg, normal distribution assumption). Alternately, if case distribution assumptions are violated, parametric tests may not yield valid results and nonparametric approaches may be preferred.

BIBLIOGRAPHY

Skrepnek GH. The contrast and convergence of Bayesian and frequentist statistical approaches in pharmacoeconomic analysis. *Pharmacoeconomics*. 2007;25:649-664.

Berger ML, Bingefors K, Hedblom EC, et al. *Health Care Cost, Quality, and Outcomes: ISPOR Book of Terms*. Lawrenceville, NJ: ISPOR; 2003.

Johnson ML, Crown W, Martin BC, et al. Good research practices for comparative effectiveness research: analytic methods to improve causal inference from nonrandomized studies of treatment effects using secondary data sources: The ISPOR Good Research Practices for Retrospective Database Analysis Task Force Report—Part III. *Value Health*. 2009;12:1062-1073.

Analyzing 2 or More Variables

BRIEF DEFINITON

The analysis of 2 or more variables with a statistical test is referred to as a bivariate test and thereby different from univariate and multivariate statistics.

EXPLANATION

Summary analysis of 2 variables is often referred to as bivariate statistics because 2 variables are compared with the purpose of determining associations, while holding other variables constant. The analysis is accomplished using statistical modeling techniques. Various bivariate and multivariate approaches are used to test hypotheses (*see term:* Hypothesis Testing and P-values) and they differ based on the characteristics of the outcome variable tested. The testing of a hypothesis comparing 2 or more groups on some continuous variable (*see term:* Available Variables for Analyses: Continuous) can be achieved through the use of a variety of parametric and nonparametric tests (*see term:* Hypothesis Testing and P-values).

VALUE AND USE

Bivariate tests provide information that allows for the interpretation of a direction and relationship between the 2 variables.

ISSUES

Bivariate tests can be misleading as they do not address omitted variable bias and confounding, the role other variables may play in explaining the relationship between the 2 variables. Multivariable analysis in the form of regression methods is suggested to adjust for the effect of the relationship between the independent variable of interest and the dependent variable.

BIBLIOGRAPHY

Wooldridge JM. *Introductory Econometrics: A Modern Approach*. 2nd ed. Cincinnati, OH: South-Western College Pub; 2002.

Munro BH. *Statistical Methods for Health Care Research.* 4th ed. Philadelphia, PA: Lippincott Williams & Wilkins; 2000.

Student's T-tests

BRIEF DEFINITION

The Student's t-test is often used to compare the difference in means between 2 independent groups on some continuous dependent variable.

EXPLANATION

The purpose of the Student's t-test is to determine whether or not 2 groups have a statistically significant difference in means. Therefore the t-test helps in calculating the probability of committing a type I error (wrongly rejecting the null hypothesis that there is no difference in means between the 2 groups) (*see term:* Multiplicity Adjustments). The t value can be calculated by dividing the difference between the sample and population mean by the standard error.

VALUE AND USE

The Student's t-test is a useful hypothesis testing mechanism when the population is normally distributed (bell curve). The Student's t-test is also a valuable tool for hypothesis testing when the sample size is small (*see terms:* Statistical Inference and Hypothesis Testing; Available Variables for Analyses). Furthermore, understanding the basics of the t-test will make it easier to comprehend the underlying logic of other hypothesis testing instruments.

The t-test can be used for various test scenarios:

- A 1-sample location test of whether or not the mean of a normally distributed population has a value specified in a null hypothesis.
- A 2-sample location test of the null hypothesis that the means of 2 normally distributed populations are equal.
- A test of the null hypothesis that the difference between 2 responses measured on the same statistical unit has a mean value of zero.

ISSUES

The Student's t-test has some assumptions that, if violated, can render the results invalid. For one, the t-test is a parametric test which means that it assumes a normal distribution. If the distribution is not normal, nonparametric approaches to testing significance should be considered. The t-test also requires a reasonable sample size.

BIBLIOGRAPHY

Wooldridge JM. *Introductory Econometrics: A Modern Approach.* 2nd ed. Cincinnati, OH: South-Western College Pub; 2002.

Wilcoxon Rank-Sum Test

BRIEF DEFINITION

The Wilcoxon Rank-Sum test is often used to compare the difference in medians between 2 independent groups on some continuous dependent variable (*see term:* Available Variables for Analyses).

EXPLANATION

The Wilcoxon Rank-Sum test is a nonparametric test used to make comparisons between subjects from 2 independent samples. Therefore, it can serve as a substitution for the t-test when the data is not normally distributed. This test can be used to compare the medians for continuous variables. In this case, the null hypothesis is that there is no difference in the median distributions for the 2 groups being compared. The Wilcoxon Rank-Sum test is calculated by first combining the data and listing, from smallest to largest, the data values from both samples. Then a rank is assigned to each value with 1 assigned to the smallest value. In the case of a tie (more than 1 observation with the same value), the average of the ranks for the tied observations are used. Finally, the ranks for each sample are summed and the sums compared. A z-test can be calculated to determine statistical significance. For the Wilcoxon Rank-Sum test, it is assumed that the 2 samples are random and independent, the distribution is symmetric and that there are equal variances.

VALUE AND USE

As mentioned above, the Wilcoxon-Rank Sum test is useful when dealing with data that do not have a normal distribution, but are still distributed symmetrically. Because the ranks are unaffected by the distance between values, this test is also of use when dealing with observations with extreme values.

ISSUES

As with other nonparametric tests, the Wilcoxon Rank Sum test may be less powerful than similar parametric tests. This is particularly problematic when dealing with small sample sizes. Therefore, it is recommended that this test only be used when the assumptions of parametric tests are not met.

BIBLIOGRAPHY

Whitley E, Ball J. Statistics review 6: nonparametric methods. *Crit Care*. 2002;6:509-513.

Wooldridge JM. *Introductory Econometrics: A Modern Approach*. 2nd ed. Cincinnati, OH: South-Western College Pub; 2002.

Hay J. Nonparametric statistical methods. In: Esposito D, ed. *Reliability and Validity of Data Sources for Outcomes Research & Disease and Health Management Programs*. Lawrenceville, NJ: ISPOR; 2013:429-433.

Chi-square Test

BRIEF DEFINITION

Chi-square tests allow for the testing of the association between an independent variable and a categorical dependent variable (*see term:* Available Variables for Analyses).

EXPLANATION

The most commonly used type of chi-square test is the Pearson's chi-square test. There is more than one use for the chi-square test. The chi-square test for equality of proportions is used for data from more than one independent population and it tests that the variable distribution is the same in each population. The chi-square test or goodness-of-fit test examines the hypothesis that the observed distribution of a variable follows a theoretical path. The chi-square test for independence tests the hypothesis that there is a relationship between the variables being tested. To calculate chi-square, take the sum of the squared difference between the observed (O) and expected (E) values and divide by the expected value for each observation.

$$X^2 = \sum (O_i - E_i)^2 / E_i$$

The resulting statistic, along with the degrees of freedom, can be used to determine statistical significance.

VALUE AND USE

The chi-square test is useful for comparing the frequencies for categorical (non-numeric) responses to nominal variables between 2 or more independent groups. As an example, for an epidemiological registry, the chi-square test can be used to test for the association between lung cancer (yes/no) and smoking (yes/no).

ISSUES

It is necessary that a series of assumptions be met in order to use the chi-square test appropriately. All observations must be independent from one another and all categories must be exhaustive and mutually exclusive. It is also important to note that the chi-square test is ineffective for sparse data (expected value in more than 20% of the categories is less than 5).

BIBLIOGRAPHY

Boslaugh S, Watters PA. *Statistics in a Nutshell: A Desktop Quick Reference.* Sebastopol, CA: O'Reilly Media Inc.; 2008.

Hay J. Nonparametric statistical methods. In: Esposito D, ed. *Reliability and Validity of Data Sources for Outcomes Research & Disease and Health Management Programs.* Lawrenceville, NJ: ISPOR; 2013:429-433.

Analysis of Variance (ANOVA)

BRIEF DEFINITION

The ANOVA is often used to compare the difference in means between 3 or more groups on some continuous dependent variable (*see terms:* Available Variables for Analyses: Continuous; Student's T-tests). Unlike Student's t-test for 2 groups, the ANOVA can be used to adjust for specific covariates of interest.

EXPLANATION

The ANOVA procedure is one of the most powerful statistical techniques. ANOVA is a general technique that can be used to test the hypothesis that the means among 3 or more groups are equal under the assumption that the sampled populations are normally distributed, are independent of one another, and have equal levels of variation. The test score obtained from the ANOVA procedure is the F-score, which can then be used to determine the p-value.

VALUE AND USE

The value of the ANOVA procedure lies in the ability to examine multiple populations and determine if a difference exists between the independent populations. An ANOVA should always be presented together with the univariate statistics (*see term:* Summary Statistics for Quantitative Variables).

ISSUES

In order for results of the ANOVA test to be valid, a number of assumptions have to be met. As stated above, these include the populations having equal variance, independence from one another, and normal distribution. Additionally, nonnormal distributions can result in an unreliable F-test.

BIBLIOGRAPHY

Wooldridge JM. *Introductory Econometrics: A Modern Approach.* 2nd ed. Cincinnati, OH: South-Western College Pub; 2002.

Ordinary Least Squares (OLS) Models

BRIEF DEFINITION

The OLS regression models allow for the testing of the association between an independent variable and a continuous dependent variable while holding other confounding variables constant. The OLS model is the most preferred regression model for continuous variables (*see term:* Quantitative Variables), provided that all assumptions are withheld.

EXPLANATION

Within this standard regression equation, the goal is to predict the value of the dependent variable (y) as accurately as possible. In order to achieve this, each independent variable (x1, x2, x3, etc.) is given a regression coefficient (β1, β2, β3, etc.). In addition, error (e) measures the data dispersion around the line of regression. This component is accounted for as it is not expected that y will be perfectly predicted.

VALUE AND USE

The OLS regression model, unless otherwise denoted, is the regression model most commonly utilized. The dependent variable in OLS regression is modeled as a function of the independent variable. This method can be used to model, predict, and forecast relationships of variables. Of note, however, the underlying assumptions need to be satisfied in order for the regression model to be accurate.

ISSUES

Cases where the underlying assumptions fail to be fulfilled have led to criticism of the OLS regression model. Data which meets the assumptions of OLS are rare and investigators should closely observe the assumptions to determine appropriateness of the model. In addition, disproving an established model can be much more challenging than fitting a model.

BIBLIOGRAPHY

Wooldridge JM. *Introductory Econometrics: A Modern Approach*. 2nd ed. Cincinnati, OH: South-Western College Pub; 2002.

Hay J. Nonparametric statistical methods. In: Esposito D, ed. *Reliability and Validity of Data Sources for Outcomes Research & Disease and Health Management Programs*. Lawrenceville, NJ: ISPOR; 2013:429-433.

Caro JJ, Briggs AH, Siebert U, et al. Modeling good research practices—overview: a report of the ISPOR-SMDM modeling good research practices task force-1. *Value Health*. 2012;15:796-803. http://www.ispor.org/workpaper/Modeling-Good-Research-Practices-Overview.asp. Accessed April 27, 2013.

Logistic/Logit and Probit Models

BRIEF DEFINITION

Logistic and probit regression models allow for the testing of the association between an independent variable (IV) and a dichotomous dependent variable (DV) while holding other confounding variables constant (*see term:* Available Variables for Analyses).

» *Ordinal Logistic/Logit and Ordinal Probit Models*

Ordinal logistic (logit) and probit regression models allow for the testing of the association between an IV and an ordinal DV while holding other confounding variables constant.

» *Multinomial Logistic/Logit and Multinomial Probit Models*

Multinomial logistic (logit) and probit regression models allow for the testing of the association between an IV and a multinomial DV while holding other confounding variables constant.

EXPLANATION

The probit and logit models are quite similar. The probit model assumes fixed-level independent variables and a linear relationship with equal variance of the dependent variable over levels of the independent variable. Probit and logit typically provide similar results and therefore most regard the 2 as interchangeable. The primary difference between the 2 is that the standard errors in a logit model follow a standard logistic distribution, whereas the standard errors in a probit model follow a normal distribution.

VALUE AND USE

Logistic/Probit models allow the researcher to estimate the effect of a key IV on a binary outcome while holding other covariates constant. As an example for using a logit model, the possible relation between hypertension (yes/no) and smoking (yes /no), obesity (yes/no) and diabetes mellitus (yes/no) could be shown. A p-value would be calculated for each of the potential covariates to check whether or not the respective covariate has an association with the DV. This method is often used in registries to adjust for possible covariates/confounders (*see term:* Confounders/ Covariates).

ISSUES

It is commonly thought that logit and probit models give virtually identical results. While this is usually true with univariate analysis, in multivariate analysis this is not always the case. For IVs with extreme levels, the logit model appears to be a better fit. The probit model fits better with more moderate sized data sets. Also, logit models work best when the categories of the DV are equally dispersed. If the categories of the DV tend to pool toward the middle, then the probit model is often a better choice.

The logit/probit models also suffer from lack of control on time varying variables, which can be a significant issue when trying to determine the association between exposure and outcome in a registry.

BIBLIOGRAPHY

Wooldridge JM. *Introductory Econometrics: A Modern Approach.* 2nd ed. Cincinnati, OH: South-Western College Pub; 2002.

Hay J. Nonparametric statistical methods. In: Esposito D, ed. *Reliability and Validity of Data Sources for Outcomes Research & Disease and Health Management Programs.* Lawrenceville, NJ: ISPOR; 2013:429-433.

Caro JJ, Briggs AH, Siebert U, et al. Modeling good research practices—overview: a report of the ISPOR-SMDM modeling good research practices task force-1. *Value Health.* 2012;15:796-803. http://www.ispor.org/workpaper/Modeling-Good-Research-Practices-Overview.asp. Accessed April 27, 2013.

Poisson Model

BRIEF DEFINITION

Poisson regression models allow for the testing of the association between an IV and a DV categorized as a rate or count while holding other confounding variables constant.

EXPLANATION

The Poisson model tracks occurrences of an event over a given quantity (ie, distance, time, area, etc.). The mean can then be determined as the average number of the events, given all events occur within the same unit of measurement. All intervals of measurement occur independently of one another.

VALUE AND USE

Poisson models are ideal in the analysis of rates and work relatively well for count data when overdispersion is not an issue. Point estimates can easily be translated into incidence rate ratios to assess the risk of multiple events and can be interpreted similarly to risk ratios. In registries, Poisson models are often applied for analysis of the incidence of rare events.

ISSUES

One of the main issues that can arise when using the Poisson model is overdispersion. In the Poisson model, the mean and the variance are normally equal. When this is not the case, however, and the variance exceeds the mean, the model becomes unsuitable. It would be more suitable in this situation to use a negative binomial model.

BIBLIOGRAPHY

Wooldridge JM. *Introductory Econometrics: A Modern Approach.* 2nd ed. Cincinnati, OH: South-Western College Pub; 2002.

Yau KK, Lee AH. Zero-inflated Poisson regression with random effects to evaluate an occupational injury prevention programme. *Stat Med.* 2001;20:2907-2920.

Zapater P, Such J, Perez-Mateo M, Horga JF. A new Poisson and Bayesian-based method to assign risk and causality in patients with suspected hepatic adverse drug reactions: a report of two new cases of ticlopidine-induced hepatotoxicity. *Drug Saf.* 2002;25:735-750.

Gibbons RD, Segawa E, Karabatsos G, et al. Mixed-effects Poisson regression analysis of adverse event reports: the relationship between antidepressants and suicide. *Stat Med.* 2008;27: 1814-1833.

Caro JJ, Briggs AH, Siebert U, et al. Modeling good research practices—overview: a report of the ISPOR-SMDM modeling good research practices task force-1. *Value Health.* 2012;15:796-803. http://www.ispor.org/workpaper/Modeling-Good-Research-Practices-Overview.asp. Accessed April 27, 2013.

Negative Binomial Model

BRIEF DEFINITION

Negative binomial regression models allow for the testing of the association between an IV and a DV categorized as a rate or count while holding other confounding (*see term:* Confounders/Covariates) variables constant, with a correction for overdispersion.

EXPLANATION

The negative binomial model, unlike the Poisson model, accounts for overdispersion by assuming that there will be unexplained variability among subjects who have the same predicted value. This additional unexplained variability between individuals leads to larger variance (than expected by the Poisson distribution) in the overall outcome distribution but has no effect on the mean. This additional variability is conceptually similar to the inclusion of an error term in normal linear regression.

VALUE AND USE

The negative binomial model appears to be optimal for use when dealing with count data since it does not assume equal separation of data points (equal dispersion).

ISSUES

When dealing with outcomes on health care resource use such as hospitalizations for most chronic diseases where many patients have zero values, the use of other models, such as a zero-inflated negative binomial model, may be the preferred choice.

BIBLIOGRAPHY

Coxe S, West SG, Aiken LS. The analysis of count data: a gentle introduction to Poisson regression and its alternatives. *J Pers Assess.* 2009;91:121-136.

Aban IB, Cutter GR, Mavinga N. Inferences and power analysis concerning two negative binomial distributions with an application to MRI lesion counts data. *Comput Stat Data Anal.* 2008;53: 820-833.

Cruyff MJ, van der Heijden PG. Point and interval estimation of the population size using a zerotruncated negative binomial regression model. *Biom J.* 2008;50:1035-1050.

Kelly AB, Haynes MA, Marlatt GA. The impact of adolescent tobacco-related associative memory on smoking trajectory: an application of negative binomial regression to highly skewed longitudinal data. *Addict Behav.* 2008;33:640-650.

Lewsey JD, Thomson WM. The utility of the zero-inflated Poisson and zero-inflated negative binomial models: a case study of cross-sectional and longitudinal DMF data examining the effect of socio-economic status. *Community Dent Oral Epidemiol.* 2004;32:183-189.

Malyshkina NV, Mannering FL, Tarko AP. Markov switching negative binomial models: an application to vehicle accident frequencies. *Accid Anal Prev.* 2009;41:217-226.

Mwalili SM, Lesaffre E, Declerck D. The zero-inflated negative binomial regression model with correction for misclassification: an example in caries research. *Stat Methods Med Res.* 2008; 17:123-139.

Mullins P, Sharplin P, Yki-Jarvinen H, et al. Negative binomial meta-regression analysis of combined glycosylated hemoglobin and hypoglycemia outcomes across eleven Phase III and IV studies of insulin glargine compared with neutral protamine Hagedorn insulin in type 1 and type 2 diabetes mellitus. *Clin Ther.* 2007;29:1607-1619.

Caro JJ, Briggs AH, Siebert U, et al. Modeling good research practices—overview: a report of the ISPOR-SMDM modeling good research practices task force-1. *Value Health.* 2012;15:796-803. http://www.ispor.org/workpaper/Modeling-Good-Research-Practices-Overview.asp. Accessed April 27, 2013.

Generalized Estimating Equations

BRIEF DEFINITION

Generalized estimating equations (GEE) are often used to analyze longitudinal and other correlated response data.

EXPLANATION

Generalized estimating equations are commonly used when dealing with correlated data, ie, data in which observations are not independent of one another. The GEE is used to study the marginal (population-averaged) expectations as a function of the predictor variables in the model. This model looks at the average effect of a 1-unit change in the independent variable over the entire population. Generalized estimating equations assume that dependent variables have a linear relationship to the predictor variables. When using GEE, there should be a large number of clusters with independence between cluster observations (within cluster observation correlation is fine).

VALUE AND USE

Generalized estimating equations, unlike the GLM, are appropriate for use with correlated data. Therefore, GEE is especially useful with longitudinal data because the multiple measurements of the same subjects are bound to be correlated. Also, it is applicable to ordinal, dichotomous, continuous, and count variables (*see term:* Available Variables for Analysis). Furthermore, GEE can be used with both incomplete data (provided the data is missing at random) as well as unbalanced data (unequal intervals between occurrences [*see term:* Strategies for Handling Missing Observations]).

ISSUES

Generalized Estimating Equations do have some limitations. In order to obtain consistent, unbiased estimation, GEE need rather large sample sizes. Another issue arises when dealing with incomplete data. If the data is not missing at random then the results obtained may be inconsistent. This is particularly true when working with dichotomous outcome variables.

BIBLIOGRAPHY

Ghisletta P, Spini D. An introduction to generalized estimating equations and an application to assess selectivity effects in a longitudinal study on very old individuals. *J Educ Behav Stat.* 2004;29:421-437.

Twisk, JW. Longitudinal data analysis: a comparison between generalized estimating equations and random coefficient analysis. *Eur J Epidemiol.* 2004;19:769-776.

Crespi CM, Wong WK, Mishra SI. Using second-order generalized estimating equations to model heterogeneous intraclass correlation in cluster-randomized trials. *Stat Med.* 2009;28: 814-827.

Lebrec J, Putter H, van Houwelingen JC. Potential bias in generalized estimating equations linkage methods under incomplete information. *Genet Epidemiol.* 2006;30:94-100.

Seaman S, Copas A. Doubly robust generalized estimating equations for longitudinal data. *Stat Med.* 2009;28:937-955.

Zeger SL, Liang K, Albert P. Models for longitudinal data: a generalised estimating equation approach. *Biometrics.* 1988;44:1049-1060.

Cox-Proportional Hazards Regression Model

BRIEF DEFINITION

Cox-Proportional Hazards regression models allow for the testing of the association between an independent variable and the time to an occurrence of a binary-dependent variable while holding other confounding, static, and time-dependent variables constant.

EXPLANATION

The Cox-Proportional Hazards regression model is a commonly used method for survival analysis. Survival analysis assesses the time before an event occurs. It is called survival analysis because, originally, the event in question was death. Now this type of analysis is used with a variety of events. Cox-Proportional Hazards is considered a semiparametric model because the baseline hazard is often unknown but the covariates are assumed to have a linear relationship to the log of the hazard function (the ratio of hazards will be the same at all times). It is important to take into account that the observation period may end without an event occurring; in this situation the data is considered to be right censored. If the time of risk leading up to an event is unknown, the data is left censored. Censored data should always be taken into account when using this model.

VALUE AND USE

The Cox-Proportional Hazards regression model is used for time to event data. This model is useful for investigating the effect different covariates have on the likelihood an event will occur and is also used to analyze patient-survival time.

ISSUES

As previously mentioned, an assumption of the Cox-Proportional Hazards regression model is a linear relationship between the independent and dependent variables. Should this assumption be violated, significance tests will be less powerful and standard errors will be inaccurate. Furthermore, depending upon whether the hazard ratio increases or decreases over time, the risk will be either over- or underestimated. For this reason it is important to check each covariate (*see term:* Confounders/Covariates) to ensure the relationship to the IV is indeed linear.

BIBLIOGRAPHY

Allison PD. *Survival Analysis Using SAS®*: A Practical Guide. Cary, NC: SAS Institute Inc; 1995.

Liu M, Lu W, Shao Y. A Monte Carlo approach for change-point detection in the Cox proportional hazards model. *Stat Med.* 2008;27:3894-3909.

Martens EP, de Boer A, Pestman WR, et al. Comparing treatment effects after adjustment with multivariable Cox proportional hazards regression and propensity score methods. *Pharmacoepidemiol Drug Saf.* 2008;17:1-8.

Larsen K. The Cox proportional hazards model with a continuous latent variable measured by multiple binary indicators. *Biometrics.* 2005;61:1049-1055.

Hay J. Nonparametric statistical methods. In: Esposito D, ed. *Reliability and Validity of Data Sources for Outcomes Research & Disease and Health Management Programs.* Lawrenceville, NJ: ISPOR; 2013:427-431.

Caro JJ, Briggs AH, Siebert U, et al. Modeling good research practices—overview: a report of the ISPOR-SMDM modeling good research practices task force-1. *Value Health.* 2012;15:796-803. http://www.ispor.org/workpaper/Modeling-Good-Research-Practices-Overview.asp. Accessed April 27, 2013.

2-Part Model

BRIEF DEFINITION

A 2-part model estimates the continuous, nonnegative outcome variable with a large number of zero values and a skewed conditional distribution, using 2 separate regression equations. The first part is typically a logit or probit model (*see term:* Logistic/Logit and Probit models) to estimate the probability that the DV is greater than zero and the second part is usually an ordinary least square regression (OLS) (*see term:* Ordinary Least Squares (OLS) Models), where the nonzero DV (*see term:*

Available Variables for Analyses) is estimated, often by transforming into its log form and using a normal distribution. Other distributional assumptions such as gamma distribution with log-link also have been used to estimate the DV greater than zero.

EXPLANATION

In this section, the discussion of a 2-part model will be based on the following example: where the DV is in the form of expenditures for health care services and patients include nonusers of services, then the expenditure variables are a mix of zeros and highly skewed positive values, with a few people accounting for a disproportionate amount of the total expenditures. This presents a challenge for statistical modeling of data. For analysis of regressor/independent variable effects on expenditure for any single health care service (for example, inpatient visits), a 2-part model approach is frequently used that combines logistic/logit or probit regression on any use of the service and linear regression on the log of positive expenditures given the use of the service.

Typically, in a 2-part model, expenditures for a health care service are represented by a binary variable for the first model and then as a continuous variable for the second model. Typically the second model is run on the subset of patients that are predicted to have expenditures greater than zero.

VALUE AND USE

Two-part models are used to estimate health care resource utilization and costs.

ISSUES

The 2-part OLS (*see term:* Ordinary Least Squares [OLS] Models) model estimation depends upon the accuracy of the model assumptions. To interpret the estimated nonzero log-transformed health care resource utilization and/or costs, these values are log-normal retransformed using a smearing factor. If retransformation is conducted using a single smearing factor then it might drastically overpredict the utilization and/or cost, as the model assumptions apparently do not hold for these skewed data.

BIBLIOGRAPHY

Duan N, Manning WG, Morris CN, Newhouse JP. A comparison of alternative models for the demand for medical care. *J Bus Econ Stat*. 1983;1:115-126.

Diehr P, Yanez D, Ash A, et al. Methods for analyzing healthcare utilization and costs. *Annu Rev Public Health*. 1999;20:125-144.

Robinson JW, Zeger SL, Forrest CB. A hierarchical multivariate two-part model for profiling providers' effects on healthcare charges. John Hopkins University. Department of Biostatistics Working Papers. Working Paper 52. http://www.bepress.com/jhubiostat/paper52. Published August 2004. Accessed April 27, 2013.

Mullahy J. Much ado about two: reconsidering retransformation and the two-part model in health econometrics. *J Health Econ*. 1998;17:247-281.

Buntin MB, Zaslavsky AM. Too much ado about two-part models and transformation? Comparing methods of modeling Medicare expenditures. *J Health Econ*. 2004;23:525-542.

Montez-Rath M, Christiansen CL, Ettner SL, et al. Performance of statistical models to predict mental health and substance abuse cost. *BMC Med Res Methodol*. 2006;6:53.

Tian L, Huang JA. Two-part model for censored medical cost data. *Stat Med*. 2007;26:4273-4292.

Diehr P, Yanez D, Ash A, Hornbrook M, Lin DY. Methods for analyzing health care utilization and costs. *Annu Rev Public Health*. 1999;20:125-144.

Caro JJ, Briggs AH, Siebert U, et al. Modeling good research practices—overview: a report of the ISPOR-SMDM modeling good research practices task force-1. *Value Health*. 2012;15:796-803. http://www.ispor.org/workpaper/Modeling-Good-Research-Practices-Overview.asp. Accessed April 27, 2013.

Multilevel Modeling

BRIEF DEFINITION

Multilevel or hierarchical models deal with nested data where the observations may not be independent, ie, observations with units of analysis consisting of more than one level. The basic idea of multilevel modeling is that systematic and random effects are explicitly modeled at each level of the hierarchy.

EXPLANATION

In the social, medical and biological sciences multilevel or hierarchical structured data are the norm. Databases including registry, discharge, other claims data contain possible multiple levels of nested units. For example, patients (level 1) grouped or clustered within doctors (level 2), doctors clustered within hospitals (level 3), hospitals clustered within counties (level 4). Thus, the units lie at 4 different levels of hierarchy where units of one level are grouped within units at the higher level. In this example, it is possible that patients (level 1) are grouped within hospitals (level 2a) and health plans (level 2b). Such a data structure is called a cross-classified structure.

Multilevel models provide a framework for exploring differences between higher level units. This difference is important to explore in case of the presence of greater amounts of clustering where much of the total variability is observed between higher-level units. The common methods, depending on the objective of the study, to model hierarchical data are:

» *Population-Average Model*

For details refer to Generalized Estimating Equations (*see term:* Generalized Estimating Equations).

» *Random-Effects Model*

In a random-effects model (also known as mixed-effects model), the unobserved effects are assumed to be uncorrelated with the explanatory variables. In case of panel (ie, longitudinal) data, the unobserved effects are assumed to be uncorrelated with the explanatory variables in each time period.

» *Fixed-Effects Model*

In a fixed effects model, the unobserved effects are assumed to be arbitrarily correlated with the explanatory variables. In case of panel (ie, longitudinal) data, these unobserved effects are allowed to be arbitrarily correlated with the explanatory variables in each time period.

Both fixed effects and random effects can be applied to a cross-sectional dataset where each observation belongs to a well-defined cluster. In the case of fixed-effects models, only within-study (for meta-analysis [*see term:* Systematic Reviews/Meta-analysis]) or within-group (for example, within-hospital) variation is taken into account to influence the uncertainty of results, as reflected in the confidence interval (*see term:* Confidence Intervals), but variation between the estimates of effect from each study or group (heterogeneity) is not accounted for. In contrast, a random-effects model accounts for both within-group and between-group variation (for example, within- and between-hospital variation).

For example, Chan et al. (2009), used prospective National Registry of Cardiopulmonary Resuscitation (NRCPR) data (2000-2008) to estimate racial differences in survival for patients with in-hospital cardiac arrests and examine the associations with sociodemographic and clinical factors and the admitting hospital. The authors adjusted for the hospital site and hospital process variables using 2-level hierarchical models. In the models, hospital site and the proportion of cardiac arrest patients who were black at each hospital were evaluated as random effects, and their estimates represented within-hospital differences by race, adjusting for all observable and unobservable between-hospital differences.

Other types of multilevel models are empirical Bayes models, hierarchical Bayes models, and growth curve models. Some of the software packages available for performing multilevel modeling include SAS (proc mixed), STATA, MLwiN, HLM, and BUGS (WinBugs).

VALUE AND USE

In the presence of high amounts of clustering where much of the variability is between higher-level units, multilevel models could be used to explore the nature of this variability. Multilevel models are used when exploring differences between higher-level units and are useful in cases of increased clustering effects in these units. Standard multiple regression assumes that the observations are independent. In the presence of clustering, this assumption is false resulting in underestimating the standard errors. This would lead to incorrect inferences with more significant associations between independent and dependent variables than there actually are.

More recently, the applications of multilevel models have been extended to diverse areas including education, epidemiology, health policy, and health services research, among others. In addition, multilevel models can also offer health economists a valuable tool facilitating greater substantive insight into the processes generating research data and will complement existing econometric techniques. Furthermore, multilevel modeling may facilitate extension of the standard meta-analysis of clinical trial data (*see term:* Systematic Reviews/Meta-analysis).

ISSUES

Adequate statistical power for analysis may be a challenge in cases of small numbers of clusters. For example, although clinical trials are typically multicentric, it is challenging to study variation between the institutions in terms of patient outcomes, due to the relatively small number of institutions studied. Researchers might encounter challenges using existing clinical trials, survey data, or registry data incorporating such clinical trials that are not typically designed to collect multilevel data.

In addition, if there are limited observations per cluster (for instance, n=1 per cluster), then clusters with a single observation contribute only to the estimation of between-level parameters and not to within-level parameters. Thus, the variation associated with smaller clusters (ie, cluster size=1) may not be studied. One solution to this problem would be to group the cluster with a small sample size (n=1) into a smaller number of clusters with common attributes (eg, facility type, location) to obtain clusters with sample size >1.

Finally, depending on the type of multilevel model used for analysis, one needs to be cautious about interpreting the results. For example, random-effects models estimate conditional parameters (ie, the effect of the exposure given a particular cluster) as opposed to population average models (*see term:* Generalized Estimating Equations) that provide unconditional parameter estimates.

BIBLIOGRAPHY

Raudenbush SW, Byrk AS. *Hierarchical Linear Models: Applications and Data Analysis Methods.* 2nd ed. London, UK: Sage Publications; 2002.

Turner RM, Omar RZ, Yang M, Goldstein H, Thompson SG. A multilevel model framework for meta-analysis of clinical trials with binary outcomes. *Stat Med.* 2000;19:3417-3432.

Von-Korff M, Koepsell T, Curry S, Diehr P. Multi-level analysis in epidemiologic research on health behaviours and outcomes. *Am J Epidemiol.* 1992;135:1077-1082.

Rice N, Leyland A. Multilevel models: applications to health data. *J Health Serv Res Policy.* 1996;1: 154-164.

Congdon P. The impact of area context on long term illness and premature mortality: an illustration of multi-level analysis. *Reg Studies.* 1995;29:327-344.

Holmes JH, Lehman A, Hade E, et al. Challenges for multilevel health disparities research in a transdisciplinary environment. *Am J Prev Med*. 2008;35:S182-S192.

Chan PS, Nichol G, Krumholz HM, et al. Racial differences in survival after in-hospital cardiac arrest. *JAMA*. 2009;302:1195-1201.

Goldstein H. *Multilevel Statistical Models*. 4th ed. Chichester, UK: John Wiley & Sons; 2011.

Caro JJ, Briggs AH, Siebert U, et al. Modeling good research practices—overview: a report of the ISPOR-SMDM modeling good research practices task force-1. *Value Health*. 2012;15:796-803. http://www.ispor.org/workpaper/Modeling-Good-Research-Practices-Overview.asp. Accessed April 27, 2013.

Generalized Linear Model

BRIEF DEFINITION

Generalized linear model (GLM) is an extension of traditional linear models, which include response variables that follow any probability distribution in the exponential family of distributions. The broad class of probability distributions includes normal, binomial, Poisson, multinomial, gamma, negative binomial, and others.

EXPLANATION

GLM comprises many of the most commonly used statistical techniques for the analysis of both continuous and discrete data. The GLM, as popularized by Nelder and Wedderburn (1972), is one form of extension to the general linear model, where a nonlinear function of the response variable is assumed to be linearly related to a set of predictor variables. A GLM is typically specified by 2 key functions: the link g and the variance v. The link function links the mean to the linear predictor. The variance v relates to the mean, depending on the family chosen to model the data.

When analyzing any clinical trial, patient registry, or observational data, one must bear in mind the following critical assumptions of GLM:

1. statistical independence of the n observations;
2. the correct specification of the link g and variance v functions;
3. the correct scale for measurement of the explanatory variables x, and;
4. the lack of undue influence of individual observations on the fitted model.

In case of natural grouping or clustering of the data, the assumption of statistical independence of the observations is violated. In such a case, one needs to account for possible intracluster correlation when estimating the variance of the regression coefficients. Such robust standard error estimates that take into account intracluster correlation are also known as sandwich variance estimates as described by Huber (1967). Thus, the variance or standard errors will be computed for the clusters rather than the independent individual observations.

Proc Genmod procedure in SAS or GLM procedure in STATA could be used to analyze observational data. Similarly, svy:glm, a command in STATA, could be used to model survey data.

VALUE AND USE

GLM is a useful method for analysis of combinations of continuous and discrete measurements. The GLM model can be used to estimate the entire sample including zero values for observations, as zeroes in the data do not pose any problem for fitting such models. GLM may be used as the second part of a 2-part model. For example, the GLM model is efficient in modeling health care expenditure data, as it directly models the mean and variance functions on the original scale of the dependent variable (*see term:* Available Variables for Analysis). The mean costs are interpretable without retransforming the dependent variable from the log to the original scale which is typically performed when data are modeled using log-transformed dependent variable in the OLS regression model (*see term:* Ordinary Least Squares [OLS] Models). Thus, GLM might be preferred to model the log-transformed dependent variable, when modeling the mean structure is of ultimate interest.

ISSUES

A potential issue with GLM approach is that if the distribution of log scale residuals is highly kurtotic (kurtosis is a measure where data distribution is flat or peaked relative to normal distribution) and if the family or variance function is misspecified, then the GLM might produce imprecise estimates. In addition, for smaller sample sizes, GLM with gamma distribution is less consistent.

BIBLIOGRAPHY

Manning WG, Mullahy J. Estimating log models: to transform or not to transform? *J Health Econ.* 2001;20:461-494.

Wooldridge JM. *Introductory Econometrics: A Modern Approach.* 3rd ed. Mason, OH: South-Western College Pub; 2006.

Nelder JA, Wedderburn RWM. Generalized linear models. *J R Statist Soc A.* 1972;135:370-384.

The Genmod procedure. Version 8. SAS Institute http://www.math.wpi.edu/saspdf/stat/chap29.pdf. 1999. Accessed April 18, 2013.

Buntin MB, Zaslavsky AM. Too much ado about two-part models and transformation? Comparing methods of modeling Medicare expenditures. *J Health Econ.* 2004;23:525-542.

McCullagh P, Nedler JA. *Generalized Linear Models.* 2nd ed. London, UK: Chapman & Hall; 1989.

Breslow NE. *Generalized Linear Models: Checking Assumptions and Strengthening Conclusions.* Congresso Nazionale Societa Italiana di Biometria Centro Convegni S. Agostino, Cortona. June 16-17, 1995. http://faculty.washington.edu/norm/pubs/glm.pdf. Accessed April 18, 2013.

Montez-Rath M, Christiansen CL, Ettner SL, et al. Performance of statistical models to predict mental health and substance abuse cost. *BMC Med Res Methodol.* 2006;6:53. http://www.ncbi.nlm.nih.gov/pmc/articles/PMC1636059/. Accessed April 27, 2013.

Moran JL, Solomon PJ, Peisach AR, Martin J. New models for old questions: generalized linear models for cost prediction. *J Eval Clin Prac*t. 2007;13:381-389.

Caro JJ, Briggs AH, Siebert U, et al. Modeling good research practices—overview: a report of the ISPOR-SMDM modeling good research practices task force-1. *Value Health.* 2012;15:796-803. http://www.ispor.org/workpaper/Modeling-Good-Research-Practices-Overview.asp. Accessed April 27, 2013.

Risk-Adjustment Techniques

BRIEF DEFINITION

Risk adjustment accounts for comorbidities of individual patients when comparing outcomes between populations.

EXPLANATION

Adjustment for confounding variables such as differing disease severity at baseline is especially important in registry studies, where treatment assignment is not random. The following are common techniques used in severity adjustment:

» ***Charlson Comorbidity Index***

The Charlson Comorbidity Index is a validated method, based on medical record review, for classifying comorbidities that might alter the risk of 1-year mortality in patients who present with a particular diagnosis.

It is a generic weighted score that takes into account the number and severity of comorbidities. A higher score indicates a more severe burden of comorbidities.

» ***Adaptations of Charlson Index: Deyo/Charlson Adaptation, Romano/Charlson Adaptation, and D'Hoore/Charlson Implementation***

These are modifications of the original Charlson Index for use with an administrative database. Romano et al., Deyo et al., and D'Hoore et al., used diagnosis codes from New Jersey and Pennsylvania hospital discharge data, Medicare hospitalization data for lumbar spine surgery, and the MED-ECHO database (Quebec), respectively, to obtain the weighted scores.

» ***Elixhauser Comorbid Disease Adjustment Method***

The Elixhauser method allows for a relatively comprehensive definition of comorbidities that are associated with in-hospital mortality, hospital charges and length of stay. This method uses more comorbidities than the Deyo/Charlson, Romano/ Charlson or D'Hoore/ Charlson methods (30 rather than just 17) that can be applied to an administrative database.

VALUE AND USE

The Charlson/Deyo method is used to generate a comorbidity list while reweighting each comorbidity variable individually in new multivariable analyses. In contrast, the Elixhauser index can only be used as separate comorbidity variables, valuable in situations in which there are sufficient data to perform new multivariable analyses but less practical in circumstances in which there are insufficient observations to generate new models. The performance of the Charlson and Elixhauser comorbidity measures in predicting patient outcomes have been well validated with observational administrative datasets using ICD-9 and ICD-10 diagnosis codes and the latter modification performs better than the Charlson/Deyo method. In summary, severity-of-illness or risk adjustment allow for a fair comparison of health outcomes to ensure that any observed differences between the exposure groups can be attributed to the health care interventions and not to differences between the subjects included in the analysis.

ISSUES

Based on the predictive validity of the Charlson index, it may not be a useful tool to measure and adjust for comorbidity in studies focused on HRQOL outcomes (*see term:* Health-Related Quality of Life [HRQOL] Outcomes), especially for patient groups with low levels of serious comorbidities, eg, patients undergoing elective surgeries. Under these circumstances, the Charlson index may underestimate the impact of comorbidity on HRQOL. The main reason is that the Charlson index was developed specifically to assess baseline risk of mortality.

BIBLIOGRAPHY

Iezzoni LI. *Risk Adjustment for Measuring Health Care Outcomes.* 3rd ed. Chicago IL: Health Administration Press; 2003.

Charlson ME, Pompei P, Ales KL, MacKenzie CR. A new method of classifying prognostic comorbidity in longitudinal studies: development and validation. *J Chronic Dis.* 1987;40:373-383.

Deyo RA, Cherkin DC, Ciol MA. Adapting a clinical comorbidity index for use with ICD-9-CM administrative databases. *J Clin Epidemiol.* 1992;45:613-619.

Romano PS, Roos LL, Jollis JG. Adapting a clinical comorbidity index for use with ICD-9-CM administrative data: differing perspectives. *J Clin Epidemiol.* 1993;46:1075-1079.

Romano PS, Roos LL, Jollis JG. Further evidence concerning the use of a clinical comorbidity index with ICD-9-CM administrative data. *J Clin Epidemiol.* 1993;46:1085-1090.

D'Hoore W, Bouckaert A, Tilquin C. Practical considerations on the use of the Charlson comorbidity index with administrative databases. *J Clin Epidemiol.* 1996;49:1429-1433.

Elixhauser A, Steiner C, Harris DR, Coffey RM. Comorbidity measures for use with administrative data. *Med Care.* 1998;36:8-27.

Stukenborg GJ, Wagner DP, Connors AF. Comparison of the performance of two comorbidity measures, with and without information from prior hospitalizations. *Med Care.* 2001;39:727-739.

Li B, Evans D, Faris P, Dean S, Quan H. Risk adjustment performance of Charlson and Elixhauser comorbidities in ICD-9 and ICD-10 administrative databases. *BMC Health Serv Res.* 2008;8:12. http://www.biomedcentral.com/content/pdf/1472-6963-8-12.pdf. Accessed April 18, 2013.

Southern DA, Quan H, Ghali WA. Comparison of the Elixhauser and Charlson/Deyo methods of comorbidity measurement in administrative data. *Med Care.* 2004;42:355-360.

Harse JD, Holman CD. Charlson's Index was a poor predictor of quality of life outcomes in a study of patients following joint replacement surgery. *J Clin Epidemiol.* 2005;58:1142-1149.

Hay J. Nonparametric statistical methods. In: Esposito D, ed. *Reliability and Validity of Data Sources for Outcomes Research & Disease and Health Management Programs.* Lawrenceville, NJ: ISPOR; 2013:427-431.

Treatment Effect/Effect Size

BRIEF DEFINITION

A treatment effect is the average causal effect of a binary (0–1) variable on an outcome variable of interest. The term treatment effect originates in a medical literature concerned with the causal effects of binary, yes-or-no treatments, such as an experimental drug or a new surgical procedure, on outcomes. But the term is now used much more generally, including in nonexperimental studies such as observational studies or patient registries. Since it is impossible to measure treatment effects at the individual level, researchers therefore focus on average treatment effects. Effect size is the name given to a family of indices that measures the magnitude of a treatment effect. Unlike significance tests, these indices are independent of sample size.

EXPLANATION

In the language of experiments, a treatment is something done to a person that might have an effect. In the absence of experiments, such as in observational studies or patient registries, discerning the effect of a treatment can be clouded by the fact that the physician (or patient) made the choice to administer treatment (be treated) and to select that particular treatment among possible treatment options. The outcomes therefore are a combined result of the physician's propensity to choose the treatment (and/or the patient's propensity to receive the treatment), and the effects of the treatment itself.

VALUE AND USE

Measuring the treatment's effect while screening out the effects of the physician's propensity to choose is the classic treatment effects problem. In practice, simple comparisons or even regression-adjusted comparisons may provide misleading estimates of causal effects (*see term:* Analysis Techniques). This may reflect some sort of omitted variables bias, that is, a bias arising from unobserved and uncontrolled differences between the 2 groups being compared. In general, omitted variables bias (also known as selection bias) is the most serious concern that arises in the estimation of treatment effects. Both selection bias and the treatment of selection bias, and thus the estimation of treatment effect, are discussed in the subsequent sections (*see term:* Selection Bias).

ISSUES

Effect size can be difficult to estimate from the literature and even more difficult to apply to power analysis and sample size estimation. Because of the complexity of analysis and the possibility of introducing bias if multiple exploratory analyses are conducted on an *ad hoc/post hoc* basis, any hypothesis testing with regard to treatment effect should be fully defined in a prospective analysis plan (*see term:* Analysis Plan).

BIBLIOGRAPHY

Furukawa TA, Watanabe N, Omori IM, Montori VM, Guyatt GH. Association between unreported outcomes and effect size estimates in Cochrane meta-analyses. *JAMA*. 2007;297:468-470.

Chan SC, Fan ST, Lo CM, Liu CL. Effect of side and size of graft on surgical outcomes of adult-to-adult live donor liver transplantation. *Liver Transpl.* 2007;13:91-98.

Rosenbaum PR. *Observational Studies*. 2nd ed. New York, NY: Springer-Verlag; 2002.

Campbell J. Sample selection bias issues. In: Esposito D, ed. *Reliability and Validity of Data Sources for Outcomes Research & Disease and Health Management Programs*. Lawrenceville, NJ: ISPOR; 2013:400-406.

Selection Bias

BRIEF DEFINITION

Selection bias is a distortion of evidence or data that arises from the way data are collected. This occurs when sample selection involves pre- or postselecting the samples that may preferentially include or exclude certain kinds of results. Typically this causes measures of statistical significance to appear much stronger than they are (*see term:* Internal Validity).

EXPLANATION

The following are types of sample selection bias:

- Prescreening of trial participants, or advertising for volunteers within particular groups. For example to prove that smoking doesn't affect fitness, advertise for both smokers and nonsmokers at the local fitness center, but advertise for smokers during the advanced aerobics class, and for nonsmokers during the weight loss sessions.
- Discounting study subjects/tests that did not run to completion. For example, in a test of a dieting program, the researcher may simply reject everyone who drops out of the trial. But most of those who drop out are those for whom it wasn't working.
- Self-selection bias, which is possible whenever the group of people being studied has any form of control over whether to participate. Participants' decision to participate may be correlated with traits that affect the study, making the participants a nonrepresentative sample. For example, people who have strong opinions or substantial knowledge may be more willing to spend time answering a survey than those who don't.
- Drugs with similar therapeutic indications are prescribed to groups of patients who are not clinically homogeneous and these patient differences are related

to the risk of the outcome being studied (often referred to as confounding by indication or channeling bias).

Selection bias may be difficult to control without additional external data, beyond that collected as part of the patient registry. Such external data are rarely available. However, several analytic approaches to address selection bias exist, including propensity score matching (*see terms:* Propensity Score Matching; Risk-Adjustment Techniques).

ISSUES

Selection bias in health outcomes research is never completely addressed and the bias persists in some fashion regardless of the technique. There is little information available on measuring the bias removed versus remaining in the analysis.

BIBLIOGRAPHY

Stukel TA, Fisher ES, Wennberg DE, Alter DA, Gottlieb DJ, Vermeulen MJ. Analysis of observational studies in the presence of treatment selection bias: effects of invasive cardiac management on AMI survival using propensity score and instrumental variable methods. *JAMA*. 2007;297:278-285.

Scharfstein DO, Halloran ME, Chu H, Daniels MJ. On estimation of vaccine efficacy using validation samples with selection bias. *Biostatistics*. 2006;7:615-629.

Nitz NM, Jumadilova Z, Darkow T, Frytak JR, Bavendam T. Medical costs after initiation of drug treatment for overactive bladder: effects of selection bias on cost estimates. *Am J Manag Care*. 2005;11:S130-S139.

Rosenbaum PR. *Observational Studies*. 2nd ed. New York, NY: Springer-Verlag; 2002.

Psaty BM, Koepsell TD, Lin D, et al. Assessment and control for confounding by indication in observational studies. *J Am Geriatr Soc*. 1999;47:749-754.

Campbell J. Sample selection bias issues. In: Esposito D, ed. *Reliability and Validity of Data Sources for Outcomes Research & Disease and Health Management Programs*. Lawrenceville, NJ: ISPOR; 2013:400-406.

Propensity Score Matching

Propensity score matching is a method used in observational studies to balance treatment and control groups based on observable covariates. Propensity scores estimate the predicted probability (propensity) of use of a given drug or procedure in a particular patient, based on his or her characteristics when the treatment is chosen.

First, the probability of receiving the treatment is estimated using observable covariates (*see term:* Confounders/Covariates). Then individual cases and controls can be matched by these estimated probabilities (propensity scores). The effects of treatment on outcomes are then estimated using conditional regression (*see term:* Analysis Techniques).

VALUE AND USE

Selection bias is a common problem in observational studies, with the treatment group often having very different observable covariates than the control group. By creating a matched set of controls, propensity score matching can be used to reduce this selection bias and thus enable researchers to estimate treatment effects when treatment assignment is not random. In addition to propensity score matching, other methods to estimate the effect of treatment on outcomes include: stratification on the propensity score, inverse probability of treatment weighting using the propensity score, or covariate adjustment using the propensity score.

ISSUES

Propensity score matching can only match on observable covariates; selection bias can still be present if there are important unmeasured covariates. It can only be used when there is significant overlap in the propensity scores between treatment and control groups. These limitations to propensity score matching to reduce selection bias should be acknowledged in the publishing and reporting of results and reflected in the strength of study conclusions as appropriate.

BIBLIOGRAPHY

Rosenbaum PR, Rubin DB. The central role of the propensity score in observational studies for causal effects. *Biometrika*. 1983;70:41-55.

Rubin DB. Estimating causal effects from large data sets using propensity scores. *Ann Intern Med*. 1997;127:757-763.

Baser O. Too much ado about propensity score models? Comparing methods of propensity score matching. *Value Health*. 2006;9:377-385.

Rubin DB. Matching to remove bias in observational studies. *Biometrics*. 1973;29:159-183.

Rubin DB, Thomas N. Characterizing the effect of matching using linear propensity score methods with normal distributions. *Biometrika*. 1992;79:797-809.

Rubin DB, Thomas N. Combining propensity score matching with additional adjustments for prognostic covariates. *J Am Stat Assoc*. 2000;95:573-585.

Stürmer T, Joshi M, Glynn RJ, Avorn J, Rothman KJ, Schneeweiss S. A review of the application of propensity score methods yielded increasing use, advantages in specific settings, but not substantially different estimates compared with conventional multivariable methods. *J Clin Epidemiol*. 2006;59:437-447.

Petersen H, Hay J. Propensity scores. In: Esposito D, ed. *Reliability and Validity of Data Sources for Outcomes Research & Disease and Health Management Programs*. Lawrenceville, NJ: ISPOR; 2013:407-410.

Treatment Effects Models and Instrumental Variables

BRIEF DEFINITION

Treatment effects models are analytical methodologies for obtaining statistically unbiased outcome estimates for treatments in which participation decisions may be correlated with variables that impact outcomes. One way to analyze treatment effects is through the use of instrumental variables.

EXPLANATION

Instrumental variables (IV) methods are econometric methods used to estimate impacts of a treatment variable when an experimental design is not feasible and selection bias may be present (*see term:* Selection Bias). IVs can be used to produce a consistent estimator of a parameter when the explanatory variables (covariates [*see term:* Confounders/Covariates]) are correlated with the error terms.

IV models are often conceptualized as 2 separate equations: one specifies the relationship between the key independent variable and the outcome (*see term:* Available Variables for Analyses), the second specifies the relationship between the instrumental variables and the outcome. Thus,

1. Y = X1'B1 + K'B2 + e1
2. K = X1'B3 + IV'B4 + e2

where Y is the outcome; K is the key independent variable measuring the treatment effect; IV is the instrumental variable; X1 is a vector of another control variable; B1, B2, B3, and B4 are parameters to be estimated; and e1 and e2 are error terms. The IV method can be used to estimate treatment effects in an observational study.

To perform IV analysis, a variable must be observed that is both correlated with the treatment choice, and is (by itself) uncorrelated with the final outcome. An example would be using changes in cigarette taxes to estimate the effect of cigarette smoking on mortality. In this example, the probability of treatment (smoking) is estimated as a function of the covariates (including the tax), and then mortality is estimated substituting the expected treatment for the actual treatment.

VALUE AND USE

When a strong instrumental variable is present, IV methods allow consistent estimation of treatment effects.

ISSUES

IVs are often unavailable for observational studies. Weak instruments (variables that are only slightly correlated with the treatment choice) will not have much power to predict outcomes, and improperly chosen instruments will create biased and inconsistent results. Studies using IV approaches to estimate treatment effects in the presence of selection bias, thus, will need to empirically describe the strength of the instrument used in the publishing and reporting of results to allow the reader to interpret the validity of the approach in this research setting (*see term:* Reporting and Dissemination of Registry-Based Studies).

BIBLIOGRAPHY

Greenland S. An introduction to instrumental variables for epidemiologists. *Int J Epidemiol.* 2000;29:722-729.

Rosenbaum PR. *Observational Studies.* 2nd ed. New York, NY: Springer-Verlag; 2002.

McClellan M, McNeil BJ, Newhouse JP. Does more intensive treatment of acute myocardial infarction in the elderly reduce mortality? Analysis using instrumental variables. *JAMA.* 1994;272: 859-866.

Angrist J, Krueger AB. Instrumental variables and the search for identification: from supply and demand to natural experiments. *J Econ Perspect.* 2001;15:69-85.

Imbens G, Angrist J. Identification and estimation of local average treatment effects. *Econometrica.* 1994;62:467-476.

Nelson CR, Startz R. Some further results on the exact small sample properties of the instrumental variable estimator. *Econometrica.* 1990;58:967-976.

Onukwugha E, Reese E. Instrumental variable methods. In: Esposito D, ed. *Reliability and Validity of Data Sources for Outcomes Research & Disease and Health Management Programs.* Lawrenceville, NJ: ISPOR; 2013:411-416.

Jackknife

BRIEF DEFINITION

Jackknife is a resampling method used to estimate the variance and bias of sample characteristics.

EXPLANATION

The jackknife is used to reduce bias and estimate the standard error using only one sample from a population with a normal distribution. The jackknife is calculated by repeatedly recalculating a statistical estimate, but leaving out one observation each time. This creates a set of pseudovalues that can be used to estimate variance.

VALUE AND USE

The jackknife method is useful when restraints of time and money or the absence of similar subjects make it difficult to collect another sample. This technique allows replication of a study using the existing population sample.

ISSUES

The jackknife is not well suited to large sample sizes (*see term:* Statistical Significance under Large Sample Sizes). This method demands a great deal of effort due to the repeated computations required. Therefore it is better suited to smaller samples. Use of statistical software reduces the amount of work necessary for the jackknife.

BIBLIOGRAPHY

Mosteller F. The jackknife. *Rev Inter Statist Instit.* 1971;39:363-368.

Bootstrap

BRIEF DEFINITION

Bootstrap is a resampling simulation technique used to estimate a distribution from sample characteristics.

EXPLANATION

Bootstrapping is a method in which a series of samples of the same size, and equal in size to the original study sample, are drawn from the original dataset and used to calculate the intended measure. This process is replicated many times, the results of which are then used to approximate the true distribution of the dataset.

Likewise, the standard error is calculated using the standard deviation existing between the series of samples calculated. In addition, the 95% CI (*see term:* Confidence Intervals) can be approximated using the interval range from 95% of the samples. Other methods, however, do exist for determining the confidence interval from the collected samples.

One of the most influencing factors on the significance of the results is the size of the original sample. In short, the larger the original sample, the more accurate the obtained CI is. Although it is best to draw a large number of samples from the original data set as well, the CI accuracy obtained from this bootstrapping technique is still dependent on the original sample size being large.

VALUE AND USE

The bootstrapping technique is most valuable for use in health economics, namely for incremental cost distributions, which generally don't follow normal patterns.

ISSUES

In order for the bootstrapping method to be worthwhile, the original sample size must be large. There is also a nonparametric method derived from the Central Limit Theorem, which does not rely heavily on the original sample distribution, but rather, states that the pulled sample means represent an approximately normal distribution. Similar to bootstrapping, though, the Central Limit Theorem also grows more accurate with increasing original sample sizes.

BIBLIOGRAPHY

Chernick MR. *Bootstrap Methods: A Guide for Practitioners and Researchers*. 2nd ed. Hoboken, NJ: John Wiley & Sons; 2008.

Nixon RM, Wonderling D, Grieve RD. Non-parametric methods for cost-effectiveness analysis: the central limit theorem and the bootstrap compared. *Health Econ*. 2010;19:316-333.

Walters SJ, Campbell MJ. The use of bootstrap methods for estimating sample size and analyzing health-related quality of life outcomes. *Stat Med*. 2005;24:1075-1102.

O'Hagan A, Stevens JW. Assessing and comparing costs: how robust are the bootstrap and methods based on asymptotic normality? *Health Econ*. 2003;12:33-49.

Payakachat N. Bootstrap method. In: Esposito D, ed. *Reliability and Validity of Data Sources for Outcomes Research & Disease and Health Management Programs.* Lawrenceville, NJ: ISPOR; 2013:421-422.

Systematic Reviews/Meta-analysis

» *Systematic Reviews*

Evidence-based medicine highlights the importance of making decisions about prevention, diagnosis, or treatment on the basis of sound scientific evidence. A systematic review or research synthesis is a structured literature review to systematically search the literature for relevant scientific evidence on a specific topic. Studies identified to be relevant to the search are then critically appraised and synthesized according to a research question, predetermined review criteria and with an explicit review protocol. The technique provides a summary of the evidence of the research in that particular topic. A meta-analysis statistically analyses this summary of the evidence in order to arrive at some definitive conclusions on the topic.

» *Meta-analysis*

Meta-analyses are not always performed on synthesized and systematic review evidence, although they do provide a means of comparing trial data across studies, not afforded by a systematic literature review in isolation.

EXPLANATION

With the massive growth in the volume of scientific knowledge in past decades, it is practically impossible for one to keep abreast with the findings in the literature. A systematic review of the scientific literature offers the provision of evidence-based information for decision making to clinicians, scientists, regulatory agencies, guideline developers, grant awarding bodies, ethics boards and researchers. For the results of a systematic review to be meaningful, the process must be formal and based on a comprehensive search of the relevant literature.

The quality of a systematic review depends on the extent to which scientific methods are used to minimize risk of error and bias. Conducting a systematic review requires a clear and replicable stepwise process: First, formulate a clear question to address in the review. For example, does patient education in chronic disease have therapeutic value? Or are amoxicillin and folate inhibitors as effective as other antibiotics for acute sinusitis? Second, develop a search strategy and selection criteria to be used for inclusion/exclusion of studies in the systematic review and include a rationale for the selection criteria. For example, if only English-language studies are selected for the review, it should be justified. Third, search the literature. Generally, this step involves searching computerized literature databases such as PsycINFO, MEDLINE, EMBASE, CINAHL, and all other pertinent databases, which may be appropriate for finding published literature on the study questions. Additional relevant studies (published and unpublished) can also be obtained by manually searching the bibliographies of retrieved articles and reports and conference proceedings, grey literature websites and clinical trial repositories. Fourth, critically appraise the studies. Ideally, the studies should be reviewed for inclusion by at least 2 independent reviewers. Fifth, combine the results. This step produces the bottom line. The final step is placing the results of the combined unbiased selection of studies in context to the original research question.

The steps discussed above for systematic review are the same for meta-analysis with the exception of the sixth step in which the abstracted data are analyzed using statistical methods. Meta-analysis includes statistical tests of heterogeneity of the study results, estimating the overall measures of association between exposed and unexposed, calculating a summary estimate of the effect size to explore the reasons for differences in effects between and among studies, and a test of homogeneity of the effect size. Where the results are homogenous, a summary estimate of the effect size across studies (usually bounded by a 95% CI [*see term:* Confidence Intervals] reflecting the precision with which the effect size has been estimated in that study) can be correctly estimated using both the fixed-effects and/or random-effects models (*see terms:* Fixed Effect Model; Random Effects Model). Briefly, a fixed-effects model states that the results of the analysis are conditional on the populations of the included studies. A random-effects model assumes that the study results reflect outcomes in a broader population. The effect size of a meta-analysis can be computed with full or partial statistical information presented in the study. There are several software packages available today to conduct meta-analysis. Some of these are commercially available and include STATA, SAS, and Comprehensive Meta-Analysis.™

VALUE AND USE

If well conducted, systematic reviews can overcome most of the limitations of traditional narrative literature reviews by providing a more objective, comprehensive and replicable summary of the past body of literature in a given topic, identifying gaps, contextualizing new materials, and producing answers to new questions, or informing and shaping future research. Systematic reviews summarize and clarify the state of science at a given point in time and can provide a knowledge base for practitioners and policy makers who may use the findings to assess the effectiveness and detect harms of an intervention. Grant-awarding bodies and research ethics boards often require systematic reviews as justification for new research. Recently, systematic reviews have become increasingly important in outcomes research, particularly to ensure that the best available PRO instrument is used to measure a preferred end point.

Meta-analysis has emerged as an important tool in decision making in social, behavioral, and biomedical sciences. The benefits of the techniques include the ability to improve the power of small or inconclusive studies to answer questions, the ability to bring together and compare trial data, and the ability to identify sources of diversity across various types of studies. Meta-analytic findings may also lead to a better understanding of scientific progress made in a particular field and reveal how heterogeneity among populations affects the effectiveness of medical interventions in different settings and in different subgroups of patients.

ISSUES

The benefits of conducting and using systematic review and meta-analysis to synthesize the available evidence for a given question to inform policy have been recognized, as evidenced by the increasing use of these research techniques. While systematic reviews and meta-analyses are regarded as the strongest forms of medical evidence, a recent review of 300 studies found that systematic reviews are not all equally reliable. These methods can be misused easily, biased, and/or provide misleading estimates of the effectiveness of interventions. For example, many critics believe that systematic review and meta-analysis do not remove subjectivity from the process of synthesis, or obviate the need for sound compassionate clinical or behavioral reasoning. Diversity may be both a limitation and benefit to systematic review and meta-analysis. Researchers have recently called for improvements in the conduct and reporting of systematic reviews by implementation of a set of standards to guide the search (eg, the Cochrane Collaboration PICO strategy—for Population, Intervention, Comparison, and Outcome), and ensure its transparency, replicability and flexibility.

Systematic review and meta-analysis cannot improve the quality of data reported in the original studies. If data are mishandled in the analysis or simply unrecognized, the results of a systematic review or meta-analysis may be spurious. Therefore, investigators should be aware of the limitations of these methods and strive to minimize the amount of bias in their reviews. Further, many believe heterogeneity of findings to be damaging to a meta-analysis, whereas others believe that the identification of outliers in meta-analysis deserves special attention and can lead to increased understanding and new hypotheses.

In recent years, there have been some areas in which the use of meta-analysis is developing and may increase in the near future. These areas include

1. prospective meta-analysis—planning trials in the context of knowing that they will be included in a meta-analysis
2. economic meta-analysis—to combine economic or QOL (*see term:* Health-Related Quality of Life [HRQOL] Outcomes) across studies in a robust manner
3. combining meta-analysis and decision analysis—involves combining the synthesis and decision process by incorporating the estimated treatment effects from the meta-analysis into a decision model.

With limited resources available, rigorous reviews of social, behavioral, and biomedical studies are crucial if we are to meet growing demands for societal needs. Systematic reviews and meta-analyses are valuable instruments that could resolve conflicts when reports of primary studies disagree. These methods increase the likelihood of detecting small but significant effects, which may help to generate new hypotheses and avoid redundant research. Many scientific articles are published each year with a wealth of information. For this information to be useful, it must be brought together into meaningful syntheses of evidence for medical decision making and for public health policy.

BIBLIOGRAPHY

Laird NM, Mosteller F. Some statistical methods for combining experimental results. *Int Technol Assess Health Care*. 1990;6:5-30.

Mulrow CD. Rationale for systematic reviews. *BMJ*. 1994;309:597-599.

Oxman AD, Guyatt GH. Guidelines for reading literature reviews. *CMAJ*. 1988;138:697-703.

Jadad AR, Cook DJ, Jones A, et al. Methodology and reports of systematic reviews and meta-analyses: a comparison of Cochrane reviews with articles published in paper-based journals. *JAMA*. 1998;280:278-280.

Klassen TP, Jadad AR, Moher D. Guides for reading and interpreting systematic reviews: I. Getting started. *Arch Pediatr Adolesc Med*. 1998;152:700-704.

Jadad AR, Moher D, Klassen TP. Guides for reading and interpreting systematic reviews: II. How did the authors find the studies and assess their quality? *Arch Pediatr Adolesc Med*. 1998;152: 812-817.

Moher D, Jadad AR, Klassen TP. Guides for reading and interpreting systematic reviews: III. How did the authors synthesize the data and make their conclusions? *Arch Pediatr Adolesc Med*. 1998;152:915-920.

Glass GV. Primary, secondary, and meta-analysis of research. *Educational Res*. 1976;5:3-8.

Greenland S. Invited commentary: a critical look at some popular meta-analytic methods. *Am J Epidemiol*. 1994;140:290-296.

Olkin I. Statistical and theoretical considerations in meta-analysis. *J Clin Epidemiol*. 1995;48: 133-146.

Margitic SE, Morgan TM, Sager MA, Furberg CD. Lessons learned from a prospective meta-analysis. *J Am Geriatr Soc*. 1995;43:435-439.

Jefferson T, Mugford M, Gray A, Demicheli V. An exercise on the feasibility of carrying out secondary economic analyses. *Health Econ*. 1996;5:155-165.

Midgette AS, Wong JB, Beshansky JR, Porath A, Fleming C, Pauker SG. Cost-effectiveness of streptokinase for acute myocardial infarction: a combined meta-analysis and decision analysis of the effects of infarct location and of likelihood of infarction. *Med Decis Making*. 1994;14: 108-117.

Jansen JP, Fleurence R, Devine B, et al. Interpreting indirect treatment comparisons and network meta-analysis for health-care decision making: report of the ISPOR Task Force on Indirect Treatment Comparisons Good Research Practices: part 1. *Value Health*. 2011;14:417-428. http://www.ispor.org/workpaper/Interpreting-Indirect-Treatment-Comparison-Studies-for-Decision-making.asp. Accessed April 27, 2013.

Hoaglin DC, Hawkins N, Jansen JP, et al. Conducting indirect-treatment-comparison and network-meta-analysis studies: report of the ISPOR Task Force on Indirect Treatment Comparisons Good Research Practice: part 2. *Value Health*. 2011;14:429-37. http://www.ispor.org/workpaper/conducting-indirect-treatment-comparison-and-network-meta-analysis-studies.asp. Accessed April 27, 2013.

Reporting and Dissemination of Registry-Based Studies

Reporting Requirements

BRIEF DEFINITION

The content and intervals required for reporting the status of the registry or the analyses performed on the data.

EXPLANATION

Registry reporting content and intervals will vary based on the program's objectives and design. Typically, annual reports are prepared, along with a final report at the conclusion of the study. More frequent reports are common, though, and may be required to meet publication, regulatory, payer, or other needs. Similarly, report content will vary among programs. Reports typically include clinical, safety, economic, and/or humanistic (eg, quality of life) analyses, as indicated in the protocol.

VALUE AND USE

The flexibility of this reporting schedule allows the study to best meet the product's and sponsor's needs for regulatory and safety reporting, and will also provide insight into any trends that develop in clinical effect, practice patterns, or study-progress indicators.

BIBLIOGRAPHY

Chapter 13. Analysis and interpretation of registry data to evaluate outcomes. In: Gliklich RE, Dreyer NA, eds. *Registries for Evaluating Patient Outcomes: A User's Guide*. 2nd ed. (Prepared by Outcome DEcIDE Center [Outcome Sciences, Inc. d/b/a Outcome] under contract no. HHSA290200500351 T03.) AHRQ Publication No. 10-EHC049. Rockville, MD: Agency for Healthcare Research and Quality; 2010:285-304.

Publication

BRIEF DEFINITION

Publication is dissemination of study findings in manuscript form, or presentation at scientific meetings in abstract, poster, and/or oral presentation format.

EXPLANATION

Publication of original articles in peer-reviewed journals is generally considered the gold standard for dissemination of results pertinent to a health technology's efficacy, effectiveness, safety, or value. Journals or meetings appropriate for dissemination of registry results may be focused on clinical topics, outcomes research, epidemiology, or economics.

VALUE AND USE

Making results available to other researchers in the field contributes to scientific progress and reduces duplication of effort. Information regarding the comparative effectiveness of drugs, medical devices, and procedures is particularly important to make available in the public domain.

ISSUES

Failure to publish results shortchanges the contributions of registry participants (both patients and medical professionals) and may be considered unethical. Underpublication of negative results and repeated publication of positive results distorts available literature evidence. Writing and editing manuscripts for peer-reviewed journals can be time consuming, however, and other solutions for dissemination of study findings are becoming available in the clinical trials arena (eg, publicly available databases of study results from sponsored trials).

BIBLIOGRAPHY

Dreyer NA. Do we need good practice principles for observational comparative effectiveness research? The GRACE Initiative. http://www.brookwoodacademy.org/Documents%20library%20PAS/GRACE_principles_25_october_2009.pdf. October 2009. Accessed April 18, 2013.

Zarin DA, Tse T. Medicine: moving toward transparency of clinical trials. *Science*. 2008;319:1340-1342.

Authorship

BRIEF DEFINITION

An author is someone who has made substantive intellectual contributions to a published report. Authors may include individuals with a role in designing the study or establishing the registry, collecting data, running analyses, and/or writing up the results.

EXPLANATION

Contributors to scientific papers often consist of many individuals from multiple institutions. For registry studies, contributions may stretch over several years from registry conception and initiation to the current analysis. Sponsorship arrangements and contract research can also complicate the authorship picture. Publication requires all authors named on a paper to have contributed substantially to the work, and at least one author should take responsibility for the integrity of the work as a whole.

VALUE AND USE

Authorship forms for peer-reviewed publications increasingly include checklists for specifying the exact nature of each author's contribution (eg, conception and design, acquisition of data, analysis and interpretation, drafting and revision of the manuscript) as well as certifications of responsibility for content, copyright transfer to the publishing journal, and declaration of conflicts of interest. Such forms attempt to ensure all authors have made substantive intellectual contributions to the published report.

ISSUES

Despite the promulgation of authorship guidelines, practices such as honorific naming of authors (guest or gift authorship, bestowed to an individual who does not meet the requirements) and ghost authorship (failure to name an individual who has made significant contributions to the research, typically as part of a work for hire) persist. A 2002 survey by the NIH reported that 10% of research scientists admitted to inappropriately assigning authorship credit within the past 3 years.

BIBLIOGRAPHY

International Committee of Medical Journal Editors. Uniform Requirements for Manuscripts Submitted to Biomedical Journals: Writing and Editing for Biomedical Publications. http://www.icmje.org/. Updated April 2010. Accessed April 18, 2013.

Martinson BC, Anderson MS, de Vries R. Scientists behaving badly. *Nature*. 2005;435:737-738.

Peer Review

BRIEF DEFINITION

Peer review is the practice of submitting research papers to scrutiny by others in the field prior to their publication in an established scientific journal. Peer review refers to both the process of review, and to journals which require this process prior to publication (called peer-reviewed or refereed journals).

EXPLANATION

Reviewers may accept a manuscript for publication (with or, rarely, without comments), reject it with comments (indicating that resubmission after revisions responding to the initial round of review may be successful), or reject the manuscript for editorial or quality reasons without providing an opportunity resubmission of a revised version.

VALUE AND USE

In addition to technical editing by journal staff, author revisions in response to peer review may improve manuscript quality, readability, relevance to the authorship, and transparency.

ISSUES

The length of time the peer review process takes may delay full publication of important results, especially if multiple revisions are necessary. In addition, while questions can be raised by reviewers and clarified by authors, the peer review process by itself does not guarantee validity. Proposed adjustments to the process have included early editorial screening of manuscripts, double-blind peer review and open (rather than anonymous) peer review, new more streamlined approaches by open access journals, and/or inviting commentary from the general public.

BIBLIOGRAPHY

Smith R. Peer review: reform or revolution? *BMJ*. 1997;315:759-760.

Mainguy G, Motamedi MR, Mietchen D. Peer review: the newcomer's perspective. *PLoS Biol*. 2005;3:e326.

Wager E, Middleton P. Technical editing of research reports in biomedical journals. *Cochrane Database Syst Rev*. 2008;4:MR000002.

Publication Bias

BRIEF DEFINITION

Publication bias refers to selection of studies with positive results for publication, whether by study sponsors, authors, or journal editors.

EXPLANATION

The end result of accumulated publication bias is an imbalance (preponderance of positive results) in the available literature addressing a given health care question, which distorts evidence available for decision making.

VALUE AND USE

The existence of publication bias has been well documented in the clinical trials arena. Prospective registration of at least Phase II and III interventional trials is now required for publication in most academic medical journals.

ISSUES

For studies based on registry data, no such safeguards (such as prospective registration of observational research) currently exist. Selective reporting of positive or interesting results may thus be an even larger problem in observational research.

BIBLIOGRAPHY

De Angelis C, Drazen JM, Frizelle FA, et al. Clinical trial registration: a statement from the International Committee of Medical Journal Editors. *Ann Intern Med.* 2004;141:477-478.

Begg CB, Berlin JA. Publication bias and dissemination of clinical research. *J Natl Cancer Inst.* 1989;81:107-115.

Veitch E. Tackling publication bias in clinical trial reporting: PloS announces the launch of a new online journal. *PLoS Med.* 2005;2:e367.

Kyzas PA, Denaxa-Kyza D, Ioannidis JP. Almost all articles on cancer prognostic markers report statistically significant results. *Eur J Cancer.* 2007;43:2559-2579.

Overlapping Publications

BRIEF DEFINITION

Two or more publications dealing with identical or overlapping study populations.

EXPLANATION

Overlapping publications may deal with early results, updates or extended follow-up, selected patient subgroups, or may be investigating different research questions using the same registry data.

VALUE AND USE

Similar to publication bias, overlapping publications, likely those with favorable results, can contribute to a perception that the balance of the literature on a subject is stronger than it is. It is important for decision makers to consider whether or not the presence of overlapping publications is distorting the evidence available for review.

ISSUES

There are legitimate reasons for multiple publications from the same data source, but citations should always be cross-referenced to avoid confusion and, where necessary, point the reader back to the original objective of the registry.

BIBLIOGRAPHY

von Elm E, Poglia G, Walder B, Tramer MR. Different patterns of duplicate publication: an analysis of articles used in systematic reviews. *JAMA.* 2004;291:974-980.

Acronym Reference List

ACRONYM	REFERENCE
ACRP	Association of Clinical Research Professionals
ANOVA	**an**alysis **o**f **va**riance
ARO	academic research organization
CDASH	Clinical Data Acquisition Standards and Harmonization
CHEERS	Consolidated Health Economic Evaluation Reporting Standards
CIOMS	Council for International Organization of Medical Sciences
CONSORT	**Con**solidated **S**tandard **o**f **R**eporting **T**rials
CRA	clinical research associate
CRF	case report form
CRO	contract research organization
CV	curriculum vitae
DV	dichotomous dependent variable
EDC	electronic data capture
EHRs	electronic health records
EMA	European Medicines Agency
ENCePP	**E**uropean **N**etwork of **Ce**ntres for **P**harmacoepidemiology and **P**harmacovigilance
ERMS	European Risk Management Strategy
FDA	Federal Drug Administration
FWE	family wise error
GCP	good clinical practices
GEE	generalized estimating equations
GEP	Guidelines for Good Epidemiologic Practices
GMP	good manufacturing practice
GPP	good pharmacoepidemiology practices
GRACE	**G**ood **R**ese**A**rch for **C**omparative **E**ffectiveness
HHS	Health and Human Services
HIPAA	Health Insurance Portability and Accountability Act of 1996

ACRONYM	REFERENCE
HRQOL	health-related quality of life
ICH	International Conference on Harmonization
IEC	institutional ethics committee
IRB	institutional review board
ISPE	International Society for Pharmacoepidemiology
IV	independent variable
IV	instrumental variables
IVRS	interactive voice response system
LIF	Swedish Association of the Pharmaceutical industry
MAR	missing at random
MCAR	missing completely at random
MCID	minimum clinically important difference
MNAR	missing not at random
OHRP	Office for Human Research Protection
OLS	ordinary least squares
PRO	patient-reported outcomes
QOL	quality of life
RCT	randomized controlled trial
REB	research ethics board
SAB	scientific advisory board
SAP	statistical analytical plan
SCNIR	Severe Chronic Neutropenia International Registry
SDV	source document verification
SF-36	36-Item Short Form Health Survey
SoCRA	**So**ciety for **C**linical **R**esearch **A**ssociates
SOPs	standard operating procedures
STROBE	**ST**rengthening the **R**eporting of **OB**servational studies in **E**pidemiology
UNESCO	United Nations Educational, Scientific and Cultural Organization
VAERS	Vaccine Adverse Event Reporting System
WHO	World Health Organization

About the Editors

Editor-in-Chief

Dimitris Polygenis, PharmD

Vice President & General Manager, Pharmaceutical Solutions,
McKesson Canada, Toronto, ON, CA

Dr. Dimitris Polygenis is Vice President & General Manager of Pharmaceutical Solutions at McKesson Canada. He develops and oversees manufacturer strategies supporting commercialization and patient access. His main areas of expertise relate to the strategy, design, and execution of market access programs, patient registries and post-marketing studies. He also assists clients with designing health economic and outcomes research studies, direct-to-patient programs and risk management strategies.

Dr. Polygenis holds a Doctor of Pharmacy degree from the University of Toronto. Prior to joining McKesson Canada, he held a position with the Ontario Round Table on Appropriate Prescribing (ORTAP) at the Institute for Clinical Evaluative Sciences in Ontario (ICES). Dr. Polygenis is currently Lecturer and Clinical Assistant Professor at the University of Toronto and University of British Columbia Doctor of Pharmacy Programs and Board Chair of a not-for-profit educational institution. Recently, he served as Director of Health Policy for the Canadian Association of Healthcare Reimbursement and Vice-Chair of an independent research ethics board.

Assistant Editors

Diana Frame, MPH

Founder, Frame Research, Brooklyn, NY, USA

Diana Frame is an independent consultant with over 12 years of experience in evidence-based medicine research. Ms. Frame has advised companies in the pharmaceutical and medical device industries as well as academic and non-profit organizations. Her analytic work, primarily based on systematic review of published literature, informs clinical trials planning, regulatory and payer strategy, and economic models. Clinical areas of expertise include oncology, rheumatology, and cardiovascular disease.

Frame Research is a small consulting company headquartered in Brooklyn, New York, which provides clients with rigorous summaries of evidence for health care decision making. During her previous experience at United Biosource Corporation (formerly MetaWorks, Inc.), Ms. Frame guided teams of clinicians, biostatisticians, and research analysts in systematic review methods and the use of observational databases. She has led successful software development efforts using relational database, web browser, and mobile platforms. The common thread to her diverse professional work is efficient gathering and synthesis of existing data, while minimizing the subjective nature of this type of research. Ms. Frame has contributed to over a dozen peer-reviewed publications, and participates in professional society meetings both to help develop best research practices and to present original work.

Ms. Frame received her undergraduate degree from Washington University in St. Louis, where she sampled from a sumptuous liberal arts banquet and minored in biology. She holds a Master's degree in Public Health from Columbia University's Mailman School.

Kirsten Hall Long, PhD

Senior Health Economist, K. Long Consulting, LLC, St. Paul, MN, USA

Dr. Long is a senior health economist and consultant with 20 years of applied economic, clinical, and outcomes research experience. Her diverse professional career includes research positions held in provider and payer settings, where she gained substantial expertise in measuring the quality and value of health care service delivery from varying perspectives.

Prior to starting her health economic consulting firm, Dr. Long was a researcher at Mayo Clinic Rochester for nearly 11 years, where her work focused on designing and conducting trial- and model-based economic analyses, as well as observational cost, cost-effectiveness, and cost-of-illness studies. More recent work while at Blue Cross and Blue Shield of Minnesota focused on the economics of prevention–in particular the cost and potential return on investment of interventions to reduce smoking and obesity prevalence.

Current consulting collaborations are methodologically and clinically diverse, and include assessments of the costs attributable to mild cognitive impairment, dementia, venous thromboembolism, and peripheral artery disease; as well as the economic impact of intervention for Minnesotans with Alzheimer's disease and other dementias; and the clinical and economic impact of non-emergent weekend catheterization services.

Dr. Long has substantial peer-reviewed publications and has contributed to and served as a co-investigator on federal, foundation, and industry-funded grants. She is a founding member of health economic and outcomes research organizations and continues to actively serve on review panels, committees, and task forces seeking health economic expertise.

Dr. Long received her A.B. degree in economics and biological sciences from Smith College and her M.A. and Ph.D. degrees in economics from Indiana University.

John McCormick, PhD

Senior Consultant, McKesson Specialty, McKesson Canada, Toronto, ON, CA

Dr. John McCormick is a Senior Consultant at McKesson Specialty. His main areas of expertise are in clinical study design and protocol development, design and execution of health economic and patient reported outcomes studies, retrospective chart review, database analyses and development of market access strategies and risk management programs.

Dr. McCormick received his PhD in Biochemistry from Queen's University, Belfast and did postdoctoral training at the University of Cincinnati Medical Center on folate antagonist transport mechanisms in tumour cells. Prior to his biopharmaceutical consulting career, he was a researcher and Lecturer in the Department of Biochemistry at McGill University, Montreal. Before joining McKesson Specialty, John was Director of Scientific Affairs at MedecoNovo Research, a company focusing on the optimal utilization of healthcare technologies and prior to this was Manager of Operations for The Lewin Group, Quintiles Canada, Montreal where he did extensive work on market access programs and health economics.

Section Editors

Chris Blanchette, PhD, MS, MA

Research Associate Professor, Department of Public Health Sciences,
University of North Carolina – Charlotte, Charlotte, NC, USA

Christopher M. Blanchette, PhD is a Research Associate Professor of Public Health Sciences at the University of North Carolina, Charlotte. Dr. Blanchette's research focuses on assessing clinical and economic outcomes associated with the use of healthcare services for the treatment of chronic diseases. He was formerly a Principal & the Americas Leader for the Retrospective Outcomes Research Center of Excellence in Health Economics and Outcomes Research at IMS Health. Previously, he directed the Clinical & Outcomes Research division at the Lovelace Respiratory Research Institute. This included the clinical research, biostatistics, and outcomes-research programs for the institute with more than 50 employees actively devoted to research in respiratory and related diseases in six sites across the US.

Dr. Blanchette also spent time in both payer marketing and health outcomes research roles for GlaxoSmithKline and served as a Senior Researcher for the Informatics Division of the Premier Hospital Alliance. In addition, he completed a summer fellowship at the Agency for Healthcare Research and Quality in the Center for Quality Improvement and Patient Safety.

Dr. Blanchette is a peer reviewer for the Agency for Healthcare Research and Quality's (AHRQ) Health Information Technology Research study section, the Patient-Centered Outcomes Research Institute (PCORI) and many clinical and economics journals. He is a member of the editorial board for the *Journal of Medical Economics*, Current Medical Research and Opinion, and *Drugs in Context*. He is also a member of ISPOR and International Society for Pharmacoepidemiology (ISPE). Dr. Blanchette has a PhD in Pharmaceutical Health Services Research and MS in Epidemiology from the University of Maryland at Baltimore; and a MA in Sociology, BS in Psychology and BA in History from the University of North Carolina at Charlotte.

Eric Gemmen, MA

Senior Director, Medical Affairs, Epidemiology & Outcomes Research, Quintiles, Inc., Rockville, MD, USA

Mr. Gemmen is Senior Director, Scientific Affairs, for the Outcome/Real World & Late Phase Research division for Quintiles Outcome. A 13-year veteran of Quintiles, his responsibilities include directing statistical data analysis and writing for Phase IV and observational studies, designing and implementing health outcomes studies, and providing senior operations oversight to real world effectiveness and safety studies for pharmaceutical, biotechnology, and other health care clients. Mr. Gemmen works actively in epidemiologic and outcomes research and in performing data analyses to support burden of illness, comparative effectiveness, instrument development and validation. His work has been published in *Pharmacoeconomics, Disease Management & Health Outcomes*, and *Archives of Internal Medicine*, among others.

Before joining Quintiles in 1998, Mr. Gemmen worked five years at Abt Associates, Inc., where he was involved in research design and data analysis for domestic and international health economic studies for clients such as the Centers for Medicare & Medicaid Services, USAID and the World Bank. He served as the Working Group Chair for the ISPOR Patient Registry Special Interest Group that developed this book. He holds a masters in Economics (with a concentration in econometrics) from Duke University.

Shital Kamble, PhD, MS

Outcomes Research Manager, Epidemiology and Outcomes Research, Quintiles, Inc., Rockville, MD, USA

Dr. Shital Kamble is a Senior Outcomes Research Manager in Scientific Affairs, Real World & Late Phase Research, at Quintiles Outcome, USA. She has a clinical background with main areas of expertise in strategy, design and protocol development, analyses, interpretation and reporting of economic evaluation alongside multinational randomized clinical trials, patient registries, observational studies with clinical, health economic, and patient reported outcome endpoints, retrospective chart reviews, and database analyses.

Dr. Kamble has published her research in several peer-reviewed clinical, medical decision making, and health economics journals. Her work has won multiple awards including ISPOR's "Best New Investigator Poster Presentation Award." She serves as a reviewer for *Value in Health, Journal of Medical Economics, American Heart*

Journal, Pharmacoepidemiology and Drug Safety, among others. She has served in leadership roles for and is a member of ISPOR.

Dr. Kamble holds a pharmacy degree and MBA from Mumbai, India. Dr. Kamble has received her MS in Pharmacy Administration from the University of the Sciences in Philadelphia, PA, her PhD in Health Services Research from the University of North Carolina, Charlotte, NC, and earned a Postdoctoral Duke Fellowship in Health Outcomes Research from the Duke Clinical Research Institute, Durham, NC, USA.

Leanne Larson, MHA

Vice President, Evidence Development, PAREXEL International, Wilmette, IL, USA

Ms. Larson has over twenty-five years' experience in healthcare, featuring extensive work in pharmaceutical product development and marketing, and in healthcare technology and operational consulting. Since 1993, she has been an industry leader in developing and leading patient registries and other outcomes research programs, and in advancing the science and application of outcomes research throughout the pharmaceutical, biotech, and medical device industries. Ms. Larson has also worked closely with hospitals and physicians, helping them incorporate outcomes measurement within their quality and performance-improvement systems. She publishes and speaks widely on a variety of topics related to outcomes research.

Prior to joining PAREXEL, she served as VP, Strategic Development at Quintiles/Outcome, and as VP, Cancer Intelligence with Sg2 Healthcare Intelligence, where she led their Cancer Program, tracking emerging trends and technologies impacting cancer care, and working with cancer programs across the country to optimize care delivery. Prior to Sg2, she led the Registry Consulting group at ICON Lifecycle Sciences (formerly Ovation Research Group) for over 14 years, and also held positions in Ernst & Young's Life Sciences and Pharmaceuticals consulting practice, and as a Senior Health Science Coordinator in Digestive Diseases with Merck and Co.

Ms. Larson holds a Master of Health Administration from Governors State University and a Bachelor of Science in Community Health from the University of Illinois. She is also an instructor in Health Service Systems at the Keller Graduate School of Management, a charter member of ISPOR and an invited reviewer for the Center for Disease Control and Prevention (CDC).

Managing Editor

Elizabeth Molsen, RN

Director, Scientific & Health Policy Initiatives, ISPOR

Ms. Molsen works with experts around the world on task forces that develop consensus guide lines on outcomes research methods or practices. These good practices for outcomes research reports are published in the peer-reviewed journal, *Value in Health*. She has managed more than a dozen task forces developing guidance on patient reported outcomes, conjoint analysis, health economic evaluation reporting standards, and performance-based risk sharing arrangements. She is a co-author on several patient reported outcomes reports and articles published in specialty journals. In addition to the *Taxonomy*, she is a co-author and the Managing Editor of a second book: *Reliability and Validity of Data Sources for Outcomes Research & Disease and Health Management Programs*. Finally, she contributes to ISPOR media initiatives interviewing outcomes research experts, health care decision makers and government officials.

Prior to her 10-year career with ISPOR, she was practicing as a registered nurse at Doylestown Hospital in Pennsylvania. Ms. Molsen has an undergraduate degree in anthropology and history from Duke University in Durham, North Carolina.

Index

Boldface indicates primary entry.

A

absenteeism, 39
academic research organization (ARO), 79
ACRP. *see* Association of Clinical Research Professionals (ACRP)
Active Safety Surveillance, 33–34
Administrative Databases, as secondary data sources, 88
ADRs. *see* adverse drug reactions (ADRs)
adverse drug reactions (ADRs), 31
Adverse Event Reporting; Reporting Requirements, 31–35
Adverse Events (AE), 31–32
AE. *see* Adverse Events (AE)
AE definitions, 31–32
Agency for Healthcare Research and Quality (AHRQ), 13, 125–126
AHRQ. *see* Agency for Healthcare Research and Quality (AHRQ)
allocations, random, 30
analyses
  outcome, 17
  post hoc, 156
  of routine data, 65
  sensitivity, 157
analysis
  ad hoc, 155
  interim, 155
  survival, 173
Analysis of complete cases, 152
Analysis of Variance (ANOVA), 166
Analysis Plan, 137
analysis population, 81
Analysis Techniques, 149
analytic
  datasets, 124
  design, 52
  plan, 138
  variables, 119
Analyzing Two or More Variables, 162
ANOVA. *see* Analysis of Variance (ANOVA)
Anti-Kickback Statute, 113
arithmetic mean, 158
arithmetic mean and median, 159
AROs. *see* academic research organization (ARO)
assent form for minors, 111
Association of Clinical Research Professionals (ACRP), 104
attrition, 115
Authorship, 194–195

B

baseline observations, 85
Bayesian analysis, 161
Bayesian approach, 161
Bayes models, 176
bell curve, 158–159, 163
Belmont Conference Center, 59
Belmont Report, The, 59–60
benchmarking, 116, 143
beneficence, 61
benefit/risk ratios, 43, 127
best current therapy, 51–52
bias
  cost-effectiveness analyses, 38
  follow-up or attrition, 115
  nonresponse, 112
  potential for, 49
  risk of, 131
  systematic, 82
  variable, 162
biological drug products, 128
biologic specimens, 123
biologic therapy, 44
biopharmaceutical industry, 79
Birth and Death Records, as secondary data sources, 89

bivariate statistics, 162
bivariate test, 162
Bonferroni method, 143
Bootstrap, 143, 188–189
bootstrap methods, 143
Budget and Patient Registries, 77–78
budget projections, 77
BUGS (WinBugs), 176

C
cancer recurrence, 85
cancer registry data, 83
Caregivers, as primary data sources, 87
Case-Control Studies, 47–48
case report forms (CRFs), 79, 96–97
Categorical Variables, 147
causal relationships, 29, 48
CDASH. *see* Clinical Data Acquisition Standards and Harmonization (CDASH)
CDC. *see* Centers for Disease Control (CDC)
Census Databases, as secondary data sources, 89
Centers for Disease Control (CDC), 129
Centers for Medicare and Medicaid Services (CMS), 38
central database, 99
Centralized or Remote Monitoring, 104–105
Central Limit Theorem, 188
central tendency, 158
CFR. see Code of Federal Regulations (CFR)
chance, ruling out, 142
channeling bias, 184
Charlson Comorbidity Index, 180
checklists
- CONSORT, 131
- GRACE, 133
- for site close-out, 122
- STROBE, 101, 133

Chi-square Test, 165
CI. *see* Confidence Intervals (CI)
CIOMS. *see* Council for International Organization of Medical Sciences (CIOMS)
clinical and nonclinical parameters, 8
Clinical Data Acquisition Standards and Harmonization (CDASH), 90
Clinical Data Standards, 92, 100
Clinical Effectiveness and Comparative Effectiveness, 28–31
clinical effectiveness studies, 28
clinical monitoring, 104–105
clinical quality and outcomes, 19–20
clinical relevance/significance, 141
clinical research, 19–20
Clinical Research Associate (CRA), 104, 118–119
clinical settings, real world, 7
clinical trial data, 149, 177
Clinicians, as primary data sources, 87
cluster [area] sampling, 82
CMS. *see* Centers for Medicare and Medicaid Services (CMS)
Cochrane Collaboration "PICO" strategy, 191
***Code of Federal Regulations (CFR)*, 68, 103–104**
Codes of Conduct, 127
cognitive interviews, 94
Cohort Studies, 50–51
cold-deck, 152
Common Rule, 59, 63–64
comorbid conditions, 8
comorbidity, 28
comorbidity variable, 180
Comparative Effectiveness, 29–30
comparator arm, 52
Comparison Groups, 83–84
compensation for patients, 114
Compliance/Adherence, 41–42
conclusions, inaccurate or incomplete, 21
Confidence Intervals (CI), 138–139, 188
confidentially, 71
Conflicts of Interest, 69–70
confounders, unmeasured, 46
Confounders/Covariates, 148
consent of the patient, 61
Consolidated Standard of Reporting Trials. *see* CONSORT (Consolidated Standard of Reporting Trials)
CONSORT (Consolidated Standard of Reporting Trials), 131–132
CONSORT checklist, 19, 131
Construct validity, 94

Content validity, 94
continuous data, 160
Continuous Variables, 146
contract research organization (CRO), 56–57
contracting agencies, 54
contract with sponsors/ARO/CRO, 109
control group, 83–84, 184
copyright protection, 57
core data elements, 55
Core Dataset, 78, 86
Cost-Effectiveness and Cost Utility, 40
cost-effectiveness/cost-utility analysis, 40
cost-effectiveness ratio, 40
costs of care/cost-effectiveness, 35
cost-to-charge ratio, 38
cost-utility analysis, 40
Council for International Organization of Medical Sciences (CIOMS), 66
country-specific regulations, 119
Count Variables, 146
Cox-Proportional Hazards Regression Model, 172–173
CRA. *see* Clinical Research Associate (CRA)
CRF completion status, 116
CRFs. *see* case report forms (CRFs); case report forms (CRFs)
Criterion validity, 94
CRO. *see* contract research organization (CRO)
cross-sectional studies, 65
curriculum vitae (CV), 109
CV. *see* curriculum vitae (CV)

D

data
    access privileges, 57
    anonymized, 62, 72
    cancer registry, 83
    completeness of, 116
    continuous, 55
    cost of collecting, 77
    deidentified, 71–72
    gaps in, 89
    missing, 72
    nested, 175
    principles of protection, 73
    privacy, 70–71
    scope of, 55
    type of, 55
    variables, 86
Database Build, 99–100
database storage, 123
Data Capture/Collection, 93, 97
data collection instruments, testing of, 80
Data Definitions, 92
Data Domains, 90–91
Data Ownership and Access Rights, 57–58
Data Privacy and Committees, 70–71
Data Protection, 73–74
Data Quality Assurance, 101–102
Data Transfer, 122–123
***Declaration of Helsinki, The*, 66–67**
Deidentified Information, 71–72
Deyo/Charlson Adaptation, 180
D'Hoore/Charlson Implementation, 180
Diabetes Treatment Satisfaction Questionnaire (DTSQ), 44
diagnostics, and domain-based data collection, 91
dichotomous, 147
Direct Costs, 37–38
direct medical costs, 37–38
disease burden, 36
dispersion of values, 158
distribution of values, 158
documentation, of study, 123
double-blind peer review, 196
drug approval, 126
DTSQ. *see* Diabetes Treatment Satisfaction Questionnaire (DTSQ)
due process, 79
Duration of Observation, 85

E

economic analytical methods, 40
economic meta-analysis, 191
Edit Checks/Specifications, 102–103
effect size, 141, 182
Efficacy, 28–29
efficacy/effectiveness, 29
Electronic Data Capture (EDC), 97, 98–99
electronic health records (EHRs), as secondary data sources, 88

electronic medication monitors, 42
Elixhauser Comorbid Disease Adjustment Method, 180
EMEA ICH *Clinical Trial Directive*, 66
ENCePP. *see* European Network of Centres for Pharmacoepidemiology and Pharmacovigilance (ENCePP)
end-of-life support, 40
Enrollment Log/Screening Log, 116
environmental factors, and domain-based data collection, 91
EQ-5D, 40
ERMS. *see* European Risk Management Strategy (ERMS)
error variance, 97
ethical conduct standards, 69
Ethical Principles and Guidelines for the Protection of Human Subjects of Research, 59
Ethical Rules for the Pharmaceutical Industry in Sweden, 130
Ethics and Privacy, 59–65
ethics committee review, 63
EU Clinical Trials Directive, 65
EU Data Protection act, 63
European medicinal products, 126–127
European Medicines Agency's Guidance on HRQOL, 126
European Network of Centres for Pharmacoepidemiology and Pharmacovigilance (ENCePP), 126–127
European Risk Management Strategy (ERMS), 127
European Union (EU) Clinical Trials Directive, 60
European Union Data Protection Directive, 73
Evaluating and Ensuring Registry Quality, 125
evidence gaps, 29
exclusion criteria, 81
execution codes, 124
Existing Registries, as secondary data sources, 89
exposures
  and domain-based data collection, 90
  and outcomes, 49
  rare, 51
  specific, 50
exposures/treatments, 92
External Comparator, 83–84
External Validity, 23

F

FACT-P. *see* Functional Assessment of Cancer Therapy-Prostate (FACT-P)
false positives, 142–144
family wise error (FWE), 143
FDA. *see* Food and Drug Administration (FDA)
FDA's MedWatch program, 33
FDR. *see* Hochberg false discovery rate (FDR)
feasibility assessments, 156
Feasibility of Patient Registries, 78
feasibility process, 78
financial conflicts of interest, 69
Fixed-Effects Model, 176
focus groups, 94
Food and Drug Administration (FDA), 55
frequencies, 160
Frequentist approach, 161
F-score, 166
Functional Assessment of Cancer Therapy-Prostate (FACT-P), 36
funding agencies, 54
FWE. *see* family wise error (FWE)

G

GCP. *see* Good Clinical Practice (GCP)
GEE. *see* generalized estimating equations (GEE)
general imputation method, 154
generalizability, 23
Generalized Estimating Equations (GEE), 153, 171–172
Generalized Linear Model, 178–179
Generalized Linear Models with gamma, Poisson, and negative binomial variance functions, 178
General Study Design, 46–54
geometric mean, 158

GEP. *see* Guidelines for Good Epidemiologic Practice (GEP)
Good Clinical Practice (GCP), 67–68, 119
Good ReseArch for Comparative Effectiveness. *see* GRACE (Good ReseArch for Comparative Effectiveness)
Governance and Oversight, 55–58
government funding, 54
GPP. *see* Guidelines for Good Pharmacoepidemiology Practices (GPP)
GRACE (Good ReseArch for Comparative Effectiveness), 133
GRACE Checklist, 133
gross earnings lost, 39
growth curve models, 176
Guidance for Industry: Good Pharmacovigilance Practices and Pharmacoepidemiological Assessment, 128–129
Guidance for Registries, 125–126
guidelines
  inconsistent, 49
  treatment, 53
Guidelines for Evaluating Public Health Surveillance Systems, 129–130
Guidelines for Good Epidemiologic Practice (GEP), 127
Guidelines for Good Pharmacoepidemiology Practices (GPP), 127–128

H

handbook from Agency for Healthcare Research and Quality (AHRQ), 125
Hawthorne effect, 49, 104
health and disease management, 8
Health and Human Services (HHS), 59, 128–129
health authority review, 49
health care, delivery of, 37–38
Health Insurance Portability and Accountability Act (HIPAA), 70, 74–75
health-related quality of life (HRQOL), 8, 35
Health-Related Quality of Life (HRQOL) Outcomes, 35–36
health status, 35
Health Technology Assessment (HTA), 54
Help Desk Support, 117–118
HHS. *see* Health and Human Services (HHS)
hierarchical models, 175
hierarchical testing, 142
HIPAA. *see* Health Insurance Portability and Accountability Act (HIPAA)
Historical Comparator, 83–84
HLM, 176
Hochberg false discovery rate (FDR), 143
Holm correction method, 143
hot-deck, 151
HRQOL. *see* health-related quality of life (HRQOL)
HRQOL assessments, 126
HRQOL outcomes, 181
HTA. *see* Health Technology Assessment (HTA)
humans in experimental research, use of, 59
hypotheses, confirmation of, 33
hypothesis, predesigned, 76
hypothesis-generating tool, 33
Hypothesis testing, 140–141
Hypothesis Testing and P-values, 140–141

I

ICER. *see* incremental cost-effectiveness ratio (ICER)
ICH. *see* International Conference on Harmonisation of Technical Requirements for Registration of Pharmaceuticals for Human Use (ICH); International Conference on Harmonization (ICH)
ICMJE. *see* International Committee of Medical Journal Authors (ICMJE)
Implementation and Operational Considerations, 76–86
imputation, 152
incidence rate, 51
inclusion criteria, 81
incremental cost-effectiveness ratio (ICER), 40
Independent Variables, 148
Indirect Costs, 39
inducements, 114
inference statistics, 141

Informed Consent, 59, 62–63, 111
institutional ethics committee (IEC), 63–64
Institutional or Organizational Databases, as secondary data sources, 88
institutional review board (IRB), 63
Institutional Review Board/Ethical Committee Approval, 64–65
instructions, written, 79
Instrument or Scale Validation, 93–96
interactive voice response system (IVRS), 98
Interim Analysis, 155–156
Internal Comparators, 83–84
Internal Validity, 22
International Committee of Medical Journal Authors (ICMJE), 63–64
International Conference on Harmonisation of Technical Requirements for Registration of Pharmaceuticals for Human Use (ICH), 31
International Conference on Harmonization (ICH), 66, 67–68
International Guidelines for Ethical Review of Epidemiological Studies, 66
international quality standards, 67
International Society for Pharmacoeconomics and Outcomes Research (ISPOR), 2–3
International Society for Pharmacoepidemiology (ISPE), 127
Interpretability/Clinical Meaningfulness, 95
interval estimation, 145
interventional studies, 48–49
investigational products, 79
investigational treatments, 59
investigator compliance, 124
investigator errors, 93
Investigator Meetings, 109–110
(IRB). *see* institutional review board (IRB)
IRB approval, 109
ISPE, 127
ISPOR. *see* International Society for Pharmacoeconomics and Outcomes Research (ISPOR)
IVRS. *see* interactive voice response system (IVRS)

J
Jacknife, 187
Justice, 62

K
kurtosis, 178

L
laparoscopic surgery, 44
Last Observation Carried Forward (LOCF), 152
linguistic transliteration, 44
location test, 163
LOCF. *see* Last Observation Carried Forward (LOCF)
Logistic/Logit and Probit Models, 167–169
Loss to Follow-up, 114–115

M
Matched Control, 84
(MCID). *see* minimum clinically important difference (MCID)
measurement reliability, 92
MED-ECHO database, 180
median, 158
Medical Charts, as secondary data sources, 88
medical devices, and safety, 31
medical licenses, copies of, 109
medical review board, 63–64
medication, and non compliance, 41–42
medications, concomitant, 8, 28
MedWatch, 108
meta-analysis, 189
methods of patient recruitment, 110–111
Methods section, 26
minimum clinically important difference (MCID), 142
Missing at Random (MAR), 150
Missing Completely at Random (MCAR), 150
Missing Not at Random (MNAR), 151
Missing Observations, 150–151
mixed models, 153
MLwiN, 176
mode, 159

Modes of Administration, 97–98
morbidity, 27–28, 35
mortality, 27–28, 35
Multilevel Modeling, 175–178
multimode data collection, 97
Multinomial Logistic/Logit models, 168
Multinomial Probit models, 168
multiple imputations, 152–153
Multiplicity Adjustments, 142–146
multistage sampling, 82
multivariable analysis, 162
multivariate structure, 143, 162

N

National Health Service (NHS), 55
National Pharmaceutical Council, 133
National Registry of Cardiopulmonary Resuscitation (NRCPR), 176
naturalistic studies, 49
Negative Binomial Model, 170–171
nested data, 175
NHS. *see* National Health Service (NHS)
nominal data, 160
Nominal/Qualitative/Dichotomous Variables, 147
nominal variables, 165
nonclinical issues, 118
noninferiority and equivalence trials, 131
Noninterventional/Observational Studies, 49
noninterventional studies, 130
nonmedical costs, 37–38
nonparametric tests, 162
nonrandom sampling, 82
nonresponse bias, 112
null hypothesis, 140–141
Nuremburg Code, 59
Nurses' Health Study, 50

O

objectives
  commercial, 17
  scientific, 17
  specific, 17–18
observational studies
  noninterventional, 49
  postmarketing, 7–8
  retrospective and prospective, value of, 46
odds ratio, 48
OLS regression model, 179
On-site Monitoring, 103–104
operational conduct of the registry/study, 79
Ordinal Logistic (Logit), 168
Ordinal Logistic/Logit models, 168
Ordinal Probit models, 168
Ordinary Least Squares (OLS) Models, 166–167
outcome(s)
  biomedical (clinical), 27–28
  clinical, 46
  and domain-based data collection, 90
  economic, 35, 46
  of interest, 7
  multiple, 51
  objective clinical, 44
  patient reported, 8
  perceived treatment, 44
  real-world, 8
Outcomes/End Points, 27–45
***Outcome(s) of Interest*, 147**
Overlapping Publications, 197
Oviedo Convention, 66
ownership claims to health information, 57

P

parameters, alterations of, 157
parametric tests, 7, 161, 162
Passive Safety Surveillance, 32–33
password protected files, 73
patient adherence, 35, 41–42
patient diaries, 42
patient discontinuation processes, 108
patient eligibility criteria, 108
patient enrollment and follow-up procedures, 108
Patient Honoraria, 114
patient incentives, 112
patient-inclusion criteria, 7
patient interviews, 94
patient outreach, 112
Patient Recruitment, 110–111
Patient Registries, Uses of, 10t–12t
patient registry data, linkages to, 72

patient reported outcomes (PROs), 27–28, 35, 44
Patient Retention, 111–112
patients, and domain-based data collection, 90
Patients, as primary data sources, 87
patient-satisfaction assessments, 8
patient self-assessment, 36
patient societies, 54
patient's perspective, 36
patient-survival time, 173
pattern-mixture models, 153–154
Pearson's chi-square test, 165
Peer Review, 195–196
peer-reviewed journals, 194
percentages, 160
permutation method, 143
Persistence, 43
personal health information (PHI), 71–72
perspectives, variety of, 46
Pharmacists, as primary data sources, 87
pharmacoepidemiological studies, 127
pharmacoepidemiologic research, 127–128
pharmacoepidemiology, 127
pharmacovigilance studies, 127
PHI. *see* personal health information (PHI)
Poisson Model, 169–170
policies, written, 79
Population-Average Model, 175
***Post Hoc* Analyses, 156**
postmarketing AE reporting, 32
pragmatic trials, 131
pre- or post-tests, 23
presenteeism, 39
Pretesting/Pilot testing, 80–81
Primary Data Sources, 87–88
Primary Stakeholder(s), 54
Privacy Rule, 74–75
Probit Models and Logit Models, 168
procedures, and safety, 31
PROC GENMOD, 153
PROC MIXED or PROC NLMIXED, 153
PROC MULTTEST, 144
product registry, 69
professional societies, 54
PRO instruments, 93
Propensity Score Matching, 184–185
property rights of health information, 57
PROs. *see* patient reported outcomes (PROs)
Prospective Interventional Studies, 48–50
prospective meta-analysis, 191
providers, and domain-based data collection, 91
psychometric properties, 44
psychometrics, 36
psychometric validation, 93
Publication, 193–194
Publication Bias, 69, 196–197
public health surveillance system, 129
P-values, 140–141

Q

QALY. *see* quality adjusted life year (QALY)
qualitative studies, 94
Qualitative Variables, 160
quality adjusted life year (QALY), 40
quality assurance, 17
quality assurance plan, 101
quality checks, 101
quality control systems, 79
Quantitative Variables, 146
Query Resolution, 120–121
Quintiles Outcome, 133

R

random allocations, 30
random-effects model, 176
randomization
  absence of, 49
  lack of, 46
randomized controlled trials (RCT), 7
random sampling, 82
range of values, 139
rare diseases, etiology of, 48
rationale for conducting registry studies, 18–19
real-world care, 51–52
re-analysis, 123
recall bias, 48, 97
record retention, 124
Record Retention and Database Archiving, 123–124

Recruitment and Retention Tools, 112–113
re-editing, 123
registries
creating, 54
defined, 7
fixed length or open-ended, 85
funding, 54
importance of, 2–3
objectives of, 17
real-world, 8
reasons for creating, 18
sponsors of, 54
Registries with Randomized Controlled Trials (RCTs), Comparison of, 9t
registry
credibility of, 56
design and management of, 77
governance, 55–56
oversight, 55
protocol, 32, 63–64, 81
quality of, 56
registry-based studies, a
registry budget, 77
registry data, 149
Registry of Patient Registries (RoPR), 13
registry parameters, 92
registry protocol, 108
Registry Purpose, 17–27
registry-specific SOPs, 80
regulations, inconsistent, 49
regulators, 54
Regulatory Documents, 109
reimbursement committees, 54
reimbursement rates, 80, 113
relative risk, 48, 51
Reliability, 94
Reporting and Dissemination of Registry-based Studies, 186
Reporting of Safety Outcomes, 34–35
Reporting Requirements, 193
Reproducibility, 26
requirements for participation, 107
resampling methods, 187
research funding, prioritization of, 37–38
Research Participants, 19–20
Research Questions, 20
Respect for Persons, 60
Responsiveness of PRO instruments, 95
retrospective chart review, 63
Retrospective Database Studies, 46
Risk Adjustment Techniques, 180–181
risk-benefit profile, 109
risks and benefits, assessment of, 59
Romano/Charlson Adaptation, 180
RoPR. *see* Registry of Patient Registries (RoPR)

S

SAB. *see* Scientific Advisory Board (SAB)
Safety, 31
safety-event reporting, 108
Safety Outcomes, Reporting of, 34–35
safety reporting, components of, 34–35
sample sizes, 187
Sampling, 82–83
sanctions, imposing, 79
scaling factor, 139
scatter plot, 148
Scientific Advisory Board (SAB), 56–57
Scientific Objectives, 17–18
SCNIR. *see* Severe Chronic Neutropenia International Registry (SCNIR)
SDV. *see* Source Document Verification (SDV)
secondary contact information, 115
Secondary Data Sources, 88–90
Secondary Stakeholders, 54–55
secured files, 73
SEER. *see* Surveillance Epidemiology and End Results (SEER)
Selection Bias, 81, 182, 183–184
selection models, 154
self-selection bias, 182
SEM. *see* standard error of the mean (SEM)
Sensitivity Analyses, 156–157
Severe Chronic Neutropenia International Registry (SCNIR), 149
signal-detection methods, 33
Single imputation, 152
Site Close-out, 122
Site Identification and Recruitment, 106–107
site manager, 118

Site Reimbursement, 113–114
Site Start-up, 107–108
Site Training, 109
situation-specific alterations, 43
Size and Patient Registries, 76–77
snowball sampling, 82
Society for Clinical Research Associates (SoCRA), 104
SoCRA. *see* Society for Clinical Research Associates (SoCRA)
SOPs. *see* standard operating procedures (SOPs)
source-data verification, 101
Source Document Verification (SDV), 119–120
sponsor organizations, 55
spread of values, 158
Stakeholders, 54–58
standard deviation, 139
standard error of the mean (SEM), 159
Standard of Care, 52
standard operating procedures (SOPs), 78
STATA, 176
statistical analysis plan (SAP), 101
Statistical Inference and Hypothesis Testing, 138
Statistical Inference and Tests, 161–162
statistically significant, 140
statistical modeling, 162
Statistical Significance Under Large Sample Sizes, 141–142
statistical validation, 93
statisticians, conservative, 145
statistics
  descriptive, 160
  inferential, 161
Strategies for Handling Missing Observations, 151–154
strategies when data is missing at random, 154
strategies when data is missing completely at random, 152
strategies when data is missing not at random, 153–154
stratified sampling, 82
STrengthening the Reporting of OBservational studies in Epidemiology. *see* STROBE (STrengthening the Reporting of OBservational studies in Epidemiology)
Strengthening the Reporting of Observational Studies in Epidemiology (STROBE), 50
Strengthening the Reporting of Observational Studies in Epidemiology Initiative, 101
STROBE. *see* Strengthening the Reporting of Observational Studies in Epidemiology (STROBE)
STROBE (STrengthening the Reporting of OBservational studies in Epidemiology), 133–134
Student's T-tests, 163
studies, observational, 25
study archive, 123
study closeout procedures, 108
study coordinator, 118
study designs, general, 46–51
Study Limitations, 24
study participant, rights of, 67
Study Populations, 81
study protocols, 48
Summary Statistics for Qualitative Variables, 160
Summary Statistics for Quantitative Variables, 158–160
surgery, minimally invasive versus invasive, 44
Surveillance Epidemiology and End Results (SEER), 83
survival analysis, 172
Swedish Association of the Pharmaceutical Industry (LIF): Rules for Noninterventional Studies, 130
Swedish Medical Products Agency, 130
systematic bias, 82
systematic reviews, 189
Systematic Reviews/Meta-analysis, 189–192
systematic sampling, 82

T

taxonomy, 2–3
Transparency, 25, 132
treatment, patterns of, 17
treatment benefit, 36
treatment burden, 41–42
Treatment Effect/Effect Size, 182–183
Treatment Effects Models and Instrumental Variables, 185–187
treatment guidelines and consensus, 53
Treatment Satisfaction, 44–45
Treatment Satisfaction Questionnaire for Medication (TSQM), 44
TSQM. *see* Treatment Satisfaction Questionnaire for Medication (TSQM)
t-test, 163
Two Part Model, 173–175
type I error, 163

U

UNESCO. *see* United Nations Educational, Scientific and Cultural Organization (UNESCO)
United Nations Educational, Scientific and Cultural Organization (UNESCO), 66
univariate analysis, 168
univariate statistics, 159, 162
US Department of Commerce Safe Harbor Agreement, 73
US Food and Drug Administration (FDA) Regulations, 68
Usual Care, 51–52
utility measurement, 36

V

Vaccine Adverse Event Reporting System (VAERS), 33
VAERS. *see* Vaccine Adverse Event Reporting System (VAERS)
Validity, 21
validity
  internal, 131
  internal/external, 24, 49
  of research findings, 115
variable bias, 162
variables
  analytic, 119
  analyzing two or more, 162
  binary, 147
  categorical, 147
  comorbidity, 180
  confounding, 148, 156
  continuous, 146
  count, 146
  covariates, 148
  data, 86
  dichotomous, 147
  explanatory, 148
  independent, 148
  independent/dependent, 148
  multinomial, 147
  multiple, 28
  nominal, 165
  nominal/qualitative, 147
  ordinal, 147
  outcome, 147–148
  qualitative, 146, 160
  quantitative, 146, 158
  treatment, 149
  unmeasured, 21
Variables for Analyses, Available, 146–149
variance, 164

W

waivers of informed or written consent, 63
webinars, 110
weighted sampling, 82
Westfall and Young Permutation (Hierarchical Testing), 143
WHO. *see* World Health Organization (WHO)
Wilcoxon Rank-Sum Test, *164*
World Health Organization (WHO), 66
World Medical Association, 66